The
SHANGRI-LA
DIET

The SHANGRI-LA DIET

The No Hunger

Eat Anything

Weight-Loss Plan

Seth Roberts, Ph.D.

G. P. PUTNAM'S SONS

NEW YORK

G. P. PUTNAM'S SONS
Publishers Since 1838
Published by the Penguin Group
Penguin Group (USA) Inc., 375 Hudson Street, New York, New York 10014, USA ·
Penguin Group (Canada), 90 Eglinton Avenue East, Suite 700, Toronto, Ontario
M4P 2Y3, Canada (a division of Pearson Penguin Canada Inc.) · Penguin Books Ltd,
80 Strand, London WC2R 0RL, England · Penguin Ireland, 25 St Stephen's Green,
Dublin 2, Ireland (a division of Penguin Books Ltd) · Penguin Group (Australia),
250 Camberwell Road, Camberwell, Victoria 3124, Australia (a division of Pearson
Australia Group Pty Ltd) · Penguin Books India Pvt Ltd, 11 Community Centre,
Panchsheel Park, New Delhi–110 017, India · Penguin Group (NZ), Cnr Airborne
and Rosedale Roads, Albany, Auckland 1310, New Zealand (a division of Pearson
New Zealand Ltd) · Penguin Books (South Africa) (Pty) Ltd, 24 Sturdee Avenue,
Rosebank, Johannesburg 2196, South Africa

Penguin Books Ltd, Registered Offices:
80 Strand, London WC2R 0RL, England

Library of Congress Cataloging-in-Publication Data
Roberts, Seth Douglass, date.
The Shangri-la diet: the no hunger, eat anything weight-loss plan/Seth Roberts.
p.   cm.
Includes bibliographical references and index.
ISBN 0-399-15364-0
1. Reducing diets.   2. Weight loss.   I. Title.
RM222.2.R632   2006   2006041610
613.2'5—dc22

1   3   5   7   9   10   8   6   4   2

This book is printed on acid-free paper. ♾

Book design by Tanya Maiboroda

Neither the publisher nor the author is engaged in rendering professional information,
advice, or services to the individual reader. The ideas, procedures, and suggestions contained in this book are not intended as a substitute for consulting with your physician.
All matters regarding your health require medical supervision. In particular, excess weight
can be associated with "hidden" ailments, such as heart disease and diabetes, that
should be medically determined before undertaking a major change in your dietary habits.
Neither the author nor the publisher shall be liable or responsible for any loss or dam-
age allegedly arising from any information, advice, or suggestion in this book.

While the author has made every effort to provide accurate Internet addresses at the time
of publication, neither the publisher nor the author assumes any responsibility for errors,
or for changes that occur after publication. Further, the publisher does not have any control over and does not assume any responsibility for author or third-party websites or their
content.

To animal-learning researchers everywhere

CONTENTS

*Let them gather all the food of these good
years. . . . That food shall be a reserve for the land
against the seven years of famine.*

—GENESIS 41

*Curiously enough, the immense dinner of the night
before, which ought to have lasted me a week,
made me hungrier than usual.*

—*Love in a Cold Climate*

INTRODUCTION

Shangri-La? Odd name for a diet. Name of a spa, maybe. I chose it partly because Shangri-La, James Hilton's fictional Himalayan community, was a place of great peace and tranquility; and this diet puts people at peace with food. Within days after starting it, all sorts of food-related struggles (irresistible cravings, too many food-related thoughts, uncontrollable night eating) usually go away. (For examples, see "In Shangri-La," pages 90–97.) Another reason for the name was that Shangri-La was meant to be a near-perfect place and—not to boast—this is a diet with many advantages. It is simple, powerful, and does not require deprivation. It's almost as easy as taking a pill, and a hundred times safer and less expensive. I also liked the idea of naming a diet after an imaginary place.

Imaginary places are often full of novelty and hope—think Alice in Wonderland or Harry Potter. No harm in borrowing some of that.

Blog postings about the diet that appeared while I was writing it (see "The Blogosphere Tries It," pages 113–122) confirmed my choice of name. "Last week a neighbor dropped off a piece of chocolate cake and it actually went stale. I forgot it was there," wrote one dieter. "Unheard of." Many dieters expressed pleasure and amazement. "Ridiculously easy. And cheap. And effective. What hath God wrought?" wrote one of them. "I hardly believe it myself," wrote someone else in response to skepticism—someone for whom the diet was working. It was a little like being able to see the future: a glimpse of how the diet would be received.

How did such an unusual diet come to be? I think my secret weapon was that I combined three methods of investigation that had not been combined before. One was my scientific training, which made it easy for me to understand the relevant research literature. Another method I used was self-experimentation: I wanted to lose weight and tried many ways of doing so. The third method was to play reporter: to phone weight-control experts and ask them about their research. (I learned that experts were approachable in this way when I wrote for *Spy* magazine.) By themselves, none of these methods is unusual, but they are rarely, if ever, combined. For example, millions of people try various ways of losing weight, but few obesity researchers do (or at least they don't mention it): Self-experimentation is considered disreputable. Because I studied weight loss in a new way, it is more understandable that I reached surprising conclusions.

After a talk by a young scientist, Niels Bohr, the Danish physicist, said to him, "We are all agreed that your theory is crazy. The question that divides us is whether it is crazy enough to have a chance of being correct." That was a rather flashy way of putting it. In an essay in *Atomic Physics and Human Knowledge*, Bohr was more sober. "The common aim of all science," he wrote, is "the gradual removal of prejudices." It was another way of saying the same thing: The truth (that is, good science) may appear crazy at first because it does not fit our accepted views of how things work.

Everyone will agree that the Shangri-La diet contradicts accepted views about how to lose weight. In the 1980s, the mantra was *eat less fat*. Consumers were offered low-fat pizza, low-fat cookies, low-fat everything. The Shangri-La diet says you can lose weight by consuming *more* fat (in the form of flavorless oils). In the 1990s, the mantra became *eat fewer carbs*. The Shangri-La diet says you can lose weight by consuming *more* sugar, the worst carb of all. If Niels Bohr wanted to lose weight, I like to think he would try it.

1

WHY A CALORIE IS NOT A CALORIE

One of the guys said to the other, "What I don't understand is how a girl can eat a one-pound box of candy and gain 10 pounds."
— The Daily Californian

THE NOVELIST Vladimir Nabokov coined the term *doughnut truth* to mean "only the truth, and the whole truth, with a hole in the truth." This is a good description of what we have been told about weight loss by experts. What they've said isn't wrong, exactly, but it is seriously incomplete—and the missing information is very important if you want to lose weight easily and comfortably. The Shangri-La diet allows you to do just that because it's based on the whole truth—including the previously left-out "hole."

You've probably heard the phrase *a calorie is a*

calorie. Doctors say it to patients. Weight-loss experts say it to journalists. *A calorie is a calorie* is meant to convey the common belief that the only way to lose weight is to eat fewer calories than you burn. (A food's calorie value indicates how much energy you extract when you digest it. Like the mileage ratings of new cars, the calorie values of foods are measured under unrealistic conditions—but, like those mileage ratings, they're good for comparisons.) According to this idea, if a particular diet was successful it's because you ate fewer calories. The "calorie is a calorie" experts say that in order to lose weight you must put down your fork. Do whatever it takes to eat less. "Everything should be about portion size," said Marion Nestle, a professor of nutrition at New York University, in a radio interview. Anyone who says otherwise, they imply, who says that two foods with the same number of calories may have very different effects on your weight—well, that person is . . . confused.

It *is* true that in order to lose weight you must eat less or become more active—but it is *not* true that this has to be difficult. It is not even true that to lose weight you must *try* to eat less. In fact, you can lose weight by eating *more* of certain foods—and this book explains how. You will *add* foods to your diet and you won't have to stop eating anything. Unless you want to lose a large amount of weight (say, 60 pounds or more), you may not even need to make big changes in what you eat.

The Shangri-La diet is so different from previous diets and what you have been told about weight loss because it is based on a new theory of weight control, a theory supported by considerable scientific evidence.

More Is Easier Than Less

Early weight-loss diets demanded that you *subtract*: cut calories by eating less. This prescription worked so rarely (everyone became too hungry!) that the message had to change. It became: *Eat less fat.* Cut out the ice cream, butter, French fries, hamburgers, and other high-fat foods, experts said, and the unwanted pounds will come off. This advice didn't work very well either.

The message became: *Eat fewer carbs.* Avoid almost all carbs (Atkins) or avoid "bad" carbs (Protein Power, Sugarbusters, South Beach), we were told, and you'll be healthier and slimmer. Bread, pasta, even apples and bananas were restricted or forbidden. Low-carb diets work modestly well, but they are not easy to follow ("I got tired of chicken and eggs," a friend said) and rarely produce as much weight loss as the dieter would like.

With the Shangri-La diet, weight loss happens because you *add*: You add certain foods to what you eat. These foods make you feel full and satisfied more easily; as a result, you eat less overall and lose weight. The foods you'll be adding are safe, cheap, and widely available. You don't have to give up anything. You don't need to *try* to eat less of anything or to pay close attention to how much you eat.

The Truth You Know

The Shangri-La diet is different from earlier diets because it is based on new ideas. One of them is that what you eat affects your weight in two ways— one that you already know all about, and one that's the missing hole in the whole dieting truth.

What you already know is that excess calories become fat. You've been told many times that your weight depends on how much you eat. If you eat more, you will weigh more. It's true that your body extracts energy (calories) from the food you eat, and if you consume more energy than you use most of the excess is stored as fat. From this point of view, it is true that a calorie is a calorie. It doesn't matter where the excess energy (calories) came from. It will become fat. As far as fat storage goes, 100 excess calories from raw carrots will have the same effect as 100 excess calories from banana cream pie. It is also true that to lose weight (fat), you must burn more calories than you eat. All this is true, but it is a doughnut truth.

The Missing Truth

Here is what you have not been told: Food also affects your weight by influencing what is called your body-weight *set point*, a term taken from engineering. Weight-control researchers have used it to mean the weight your body "wants" to be—the weight you are when you're not paying attention to how much you eat. Your set point may be quite a bit more than the weight you would choose or the weight that's healthy for you. In spite of the name, however, your set point is not fixed or constant. It is not your "natural weight," one unchanging magic number. Rather, your set point goes up and down, partly in response to what you eat.

By varying how hungry you are and how soon you feel full when you eat, your body-weight regulatory system pushes your weight close to your set point. Your body-weight set point is like the temperature to which a thermostat is set. My home thermostat, for example, is set to 68 degrees. The system "wants" the temperature to be 68 degrees at all times. If the temperature goes below 68 degrees, the system turns on a heater, which warms the house. When the temperature reaches 68 degrees, the heat goes off.

Your weight-regulation system controls your weight in a similar way. Let's say your body-weight set point is 180 pounds. If you weigh *less* than 180 pounds, you will be hungry and think about food. The bigger the gap between your set point and your weight, the more hungry you will be, the more you will think about food, and the more food it will take to feel full when you eat. It is nearly impossible to weigh much less than your set point for a long time—the hunger becomes unbearable.

If you weigh *more* than your set point of 180 pounds, you will not be hungry and will think much less about food. When you eat, you will feel full rapidly. (See the table for more details.)

The level of your set point depends on everything you have eaten for the last several months. Some foods are high-set-point foods; if you eat only these foods, your set point will be high. Some foods are low-set-point foods; if you eat only these foods, your set point will be low. (I'll explain why in later chapters.) Other foods are in between. Your set point depends on the *average* of what you have eaten for several months. When you eat a food that is low for you (lower than your average), your set

What's My Set Point?

IF YOU FEEL . . .	YOUR SET POINT IS . . .
Ravenous. Can't stop thinking about food. Dream about it. Nothing fills you up, even a large meal. Unhappy.	Your weight plus several pounds.
Hungry. Always feel like eating. Think about food every few minutes.	Your weight plus a pound or two.
Comfortable. Hungry sometimes. At mealtime, food looks good. You eat average amounts.	Close to your weight.
Full long after a meal. Forget to eat. Don't think about food. Not hungry until you start eating.	Your weight minus a pound or two.
Stuffed. Feel like you don't want to eat for days. Your favorite foods? No thanks. Never hungry.	Your weight minus several pounds.

point goes down slightly. When you eat a food that is high for you (higher than your average), your set point goes up slightly.

When a food lowers your set point, you will be less hungry than usual afterward. You may wait longer than usual before your next meal and you will tend to eat less than usual at your next meal. When a food raises your set point, you are more hungry than usual afterward, you may eat sooner than usual, and you will tend to eat more than usual at your next meal. The quote from Nancy Mitford's *Love in a Cold Climate* that opens this book (see page ix) is an example: The dinner raised the speaker's set point. It made her "hungrier than usual" at later meals.

By raising or lowering your set point, every food controls how much you eat *later*—how much you eat of *other* foods. By itself, a one-pound box of chocolates can increase your weight by no more than one pound. But if it raises your set point 10 pounds, it will cause you to eat more of *other* foods, enough to raise your weight 10 pounds. Your body always wants your weight to match your set point.

Diets and Your Set Point

Diets are not only about losing weight; they're also about how they make you feel. If you lose weight but feel hungry all the time, the diet is no success. You are very likely to regain the lost weight, sooner or later, in order to stop feeling hungry. This is why simply eating less doesn't work for long. You lose weight, true, but you gain hunger. Your hunger grows and eventually becomes unbearable.

Diets cause hunger when they lower your weight without lowering your set point. *The key to successful weight loss is to lower your set point.* When you lower your set point, you will lose weight without effort.

The Shangri-La diet lowers your set point because you eat *more* of certain foods—zero-set-point foods. These foods are so powerful that they will lower your set point no matter where it is. Because your set point will go down, you will feel less hungry than usual, you will eat less than usual, and you will lose weight—without any struggle at all. And without cutting anything out of your diet.

Your Set Point (Continued)

Let's go back to the thermostat analogy to understand more about your set point. A heating system with a thermostat has a set point: the temperature to which the thermostat is set. Just as the thermostat's set point is flexible (I can set it to 70 degrees, 60 degrees, and so on), so too is your body-weight set point.

To sum up, your home thermostat and your body's weight-regulation system have important similarities. Both have a set point. Both have a *flexible* set point.

There are also important differences:

- You can quickly change the thermost[a]
point—by turning a dial. Your body-wei[ght]
point changes slowly, usually by no more than
a few pounds per week.

- Your body-weight set point is designed to be
sensitive to the price of energy (calories). When
energy is cheap—that is, when calories are
abundant—your body-weight set point goes up.
Hundreds of thousands of years ago, when our
body-weight regulation system evolved, this
strategy made sense. Food was often scarce, so
when it was abundant it made sense to eat more
than usual and store the excess as fat. When
food was scarce, it made sense to use the stored
energy and lose weight. However, our current
conditions are drastically different from the
conditions thousands of years ago. Food is now
abundant all the time. As a result, this pric-
ing/storage mechanism no longer works well.
Your system decides (correctly) that food is
abundant and thus raises your set point to increase the amount of energy you have stored—
but the lean years never come. The Shangri-La
diet tricks your system into thinking food is
scarce, thus solving the problem. Your home
thermostat is simpler: It isn't sensitive to the
price of energy (electricity, natural gas, heating
oil). It's not sensitive to outside conditions in
any way.

- Most home thermostat systems are "all or none." Either the heat source is on (when the actual temperature is lower than the thermostat temperature) or off (when it's not). In contrast, your body-weight regulation system varies the strength of the push toward set point (hunger) according to how much difference there is between your actual weight and your set point. A small difference causes a little hunger. A big difference causes great hunger.

- To push a cold room (for example, one that's 60 degrees) toward the set point temperature (70 degrees), a home-temperature system will do just one thing: turn on the heat. In contrast, your body-weight regulatory system will cause at least three changes if your actual weight (150 pounds) is less than your set-point weight (155 pounds): You will feel more hungry than usual; you will think about food more often; and when you eat, it will take more food to make you feel full.

Systems with set points, bless them, are *set and forget*: Once the set point is in the right place, no further action is necessary. Once you have set your home's thermostat to the right temperature, you can forget about it. It will turn the heat on and off appropriately. Likewise, when you understand how to lower your body-weight set point, that is all you will need to know about losing weight. After you lower your set point, you will not need to think more about it. Your brain will turn hunger on and off (mostly off) in such a way that you will lose weight without struggle. Without counting calories. Without carefully choosing what to eat. Without going hungry.

How Does My Set Point Control My Weight?

If you are like most people, your body-weight set point is always close to your actual weight—sometimes slightly above, sometimes a bit below, but never far away. Your weight-regulation system keeps your weight close to your set point the way a driver keeps a car in its lane: by making many small adjustments. When your weight is slightly below your set point, you become a little more hungry than usual and it takes a little more food to feel full. When your weight is slightly above your set point, you feel slightly less hungry than usual and it takes a little less food to feel full. These changes in appetite are so small and frequent that we usually don't notice them.

If you follow the advice in this book, however, you should be able to move your set point well below your current weight—quite possibly farther below your weight than it has ever been before. Once your set point is lowered by simply adding certain foods to what you normally eat, you will be able to keep it there easily, without conscious effort. When your body-weight set point is lowered, you'll notice the following changes:

1. *You will be less hungry between meals.* You will feel less mental pressure to eat. It will be easier to avoid snacking. You'll think about food less often. If you're in the habit of eating late at night, you'll likely no longer want to.

2. *During a meal, you will feel full faster.* When you eat, it will take less food to make you feel full—to reach the point where you want to stop eating, so you will eat less. If your body-weight set point is below your actual weight, you will feel full sooner than if your set point is above your weight. In other words, when you change your body-weight set point to a significantly lower weight (by following the Shangri-La diet), you'll eat the same food and enjoy the same tastes, but you won't need to eat as much food in order to feel satisfied.

These two changes usually happen within days of starting the Shangri-La diet. They will be the first signs that the diet is working.

Some Flavors Are More Fattening Than Others

One of the most unusual features of the Shangri-La diet is its emphasis on flavor. The reason for this emphasis is that *the flavor of a food controls how it affects your set point.*

We are born liking sweet foods and salty foods,

but most flavors, such as the flavor of spinach, we learn to like—as parents know. Much of this learning is associative: We come to like a flavor when we associate it with calories. As a flavor becomes better associated with calories, it tastes better. Coke, the soft drink, is a good example. A Japanese cookbook author named Gaku Homma had his first taste of Coke when he was old enough to remember it. He later wrote it tasted "like medicine." A friend of mine had his first taste of Coke when he was seven or eight. It didn't taste good. *What was the fuss about?* he wondered. In both cases, the Coke did not taste good because the flavor had not yet become associated with calories. Because Coke contains calories, as you drink it again and again the flavor-calorie association becomes stronger and stronger and the flavor tastes better and better. Here is how a restaurant critic described his reaction to cilantro: "First put off by the leaves' flavor, after repeated exposure I grew to anticipate their taste. Then welcomed it. Then craved it." His reaction changed because he ate the cilantro with food (calories). Had he eaten it alone, his initial negative reaction would have persisted.

Flavor-calorie associations are important because they influence your set point. A food with a strong flavor-calorie association will raise your set point; a food with a weak flavor-calorie association will lower your set point; a food with *no* flavor-calorie association will lower your set point a lot.

Two Foods That Lower Your Set Point

Once you realize that lowering your set point is the key to losing weight, all you need to do to begin the Shangri-La program is eat foods that lower your set point.

If we rate foods on a scale from 0 to 10, where a food ranked at 0 pushes your set point toward zero (skinny) and food ranked at 10 pushes your set point toward a very high value (obese), we might say that raw vegetables have a value of 4, and junk food a value of 10. (Later, I'll explain why junk food pushes your set point very high, and the reason may surprise you.) If you eat only junk food (value of 10), your set point will be much higher than if you eat only raw vegetables (value of 4). Suppose you eat only junk food but then add raw vegetables to your diet. This will lower your set point, because you are adding 4's to a diet that otherwise is all 10's, and cause you to lose weight.

On your old diet, you ate foods that were 10, 10, 10, 10, 10; the average value of your diet is 10.

On your new diet, you added some lower-valued foods: 10, 10, 10, 10, 10, plus 4, 4. Now the average value of your diet is less than 10, so your set point will drop.

The Shangri-La diet is based on the discovery that there are foods far more powerful than raw vegetables at lowering your set point. If raw vegetables are 4, the two foods at the heart of the

Shangri-La diet are o. Even small amounts of them will lower your set point significantly. Here are two of these set-point-lowering foods:

Food 1. *Sugar water (unflavored).* Although sugar water is sweet, the brain responds to it as if it were flavorless. Research has shown that the brain treats sweetness differently from other flavors. (For example, young children, who like few flavors, like sweet things.) Drinking sugar water is like eating food with no flavor, which lowers your set point and helps you lose weight.

Food 2. *Extra-light olive oil.* Extra-light olive oil has almost no flavor (the opposite of extra-virgin olive oil, which has a strong flavor). Swallowing a small amount of extra-light olive oil is very close to eating a food with no flavor, which, again, lowers your set point and helps you lose weight.

Even in amounts as small as a few hundred calories per day, these foods have potent weight-loss effects. In later chapters we'll talk much more about each of these types of foods and their benefits. What I hope you've learned at this point is that weight loss can be achieved in surprising new ways. While you probably haven't heard of these new methods before, they're simple, easy to adopt, and perfectly consistent with a healthy diet. You don't need to stop eating anything. You don't need to stop eating hamburgers or desserts or bread, or, for that matter, any of the healthier choices you make. Instead, you just have to start eating one or more of Foods 1 or 2 every day. If you want to lose a great deal of weight, you may need to vary the *flavors* of your food—the flavor of your hamburgers, for example. Chapter 6, "Extra Credit: Six More Ways to Lose Weight," is about how to apply the new ideas in other ways.

How much of these foods you will need to eat each day will depend on how much weight you want to lose, but you may need to eat as little as 200 calories a day or less of these Shangri-La set-point-lowering foods. When your set point becomes lower than your actual weight, you'll be less hungry throughout the day. When you eat, you will feel satisfied sooner. You will lose weight until your weight reaches your new, lower set point. And at that point, your hunger will return to normal levels and you will stop losing weight.

2

THE CASE OF THE MISSING APPETITE

This new, $3 billion-a-year industry was aimed
squarely at the age-old pursuit of getting
thin while eating whatever you want,
which, of course, never works.

—*The Washington Post* (2005),
DESCRIBING THE LOW-CARB FOOD INDUSTRY

INTRODUCTORY Psychology was the first class I taught when I became a professor. I decided to include a lecture on weight control—not a typical Psych 1 topic, but it interested me. It was an intellectual interest, not a practical one: I was thin and ate whatever I wanted. I read a stack of scientific articles to figure out what to say. Most of them were about rat experiments that had studied the effect of dietary changes on weight. I liked reading about rat experiments. In graduate school, I had done quite a few of them, although not in the area of weight control. My doctoral dissertation was about how rats measure time.

Ten years later, I was no longer thin. The scale read 200 pounds. I am five foot ten, so my BMI (body mass index) was 29 (overweight). I had lectured on weight control many times and had given my students advice based on the scientific papers I had read. Now I took my own advice and started eating less-processed food—oranges instead of orange juice, for example. The dietary change worked: I easily lost about ten pounds. This was intriguing. Maybe reading about all those rat experiments had taught me something useful.

I continued to read scientific papers about weight control. At one point, I planned to write a popular book based on my Psych 1 lectures. While doing research for the book (never finished), I spoke to Dr. Israel Ramirez, a research scientist at the Monell Chemical Senses Institute, in Philadelphia. He sent me a stack of reprints of his scientific papers, and one of them led me to think of a new theory of weight control. (For more about Ramirez's research, see the Appendix, "The Science Behind the Theory Behind the Diet," pages 141–157) The theory, which I describe in the next chapter, helped me find two new ways of losing weight: eating food with a low glycemic index (I lost six pounds) and eating sushi (I lost thirteen pounds). This was excellent evidence that there was a lot of truth to it.

I never stopped eating less-processed food, and

never regained the weight I had lost that way. I never stopped eating food with a low glycemic index and never regained that lost weight either. I did stop eating sushi after a month or so and regained *that* lost weight. At this point, I weighed about 185 pounds (BMI 26, still overweight), definitely too much. Like a billion other people, I would have liked to lose weight but could not. Unlike them, however, I had a seriously good theory of weight control—a theory that had actually worked, in the sense that it had helped me lose weight. My situation puzzled me. If I truly understood weight control, shouldn't I be able to choose my weight? If you understand how something works, shouldn't you be able to fix it? I was unable to see the flaw in this argument, which seemed to imply there was something wrong with my theory. But I couldn't find anything wrong with it.

French Sodas Expand My Theory

In 2000, I went to Paris in order to get a cheap flight to Croatia to visit a friend. Paris being Paris, I stayed a week.

I love French food. My first meal in Paris, at a bistro, was delicious. After that meal, however, I lost my appetite. For most of the rest of my visit, I had to force myself to eat. Big disappointment!

Why? I wondered. I wasn't sick or depressed or anxious. I wasn't taking any medication. I was walking many miles per day, wandering around the city. Life was normal, for a vacation—I just didn't feel like eating. Usually I ate a lot.

As I explained in Chapter 1, "Why a Calorie Is Not a Calorie," my weight-control theory emphasizes that the relationship between your set point and your actual weight determines how hungry you are at any given moment. If your set point is *above* your weight, you will be hungry. If your set point is *below* your weight, you will not be hungry. Total loss of appetite, according to my theory, meant that my set point was well below my weight (see table, "What's My Set Point?," on page 10). I had plenty of time on my walks to think about what might have caused this.

I had never before lost my appetite so completely, so the cause was probably something unusual. Not Paris: I had visited Paris and other foreign cities without losing my appetite. My theory said that food controls the set point. So I focused on food: What unusual food had I eaten?

The bistro meal hadn't been unusual. But there *was* something different. It was June and very hot. To cool off, I had drunk a few sugar-sweetened soft drinks each day for several days. This was unusual—in fact, unprecedented. At home I never drank sodas with sugar; I always drank diet sodas. In Paris, I wanted to try drinks not available at home, but the new sodas I encountered didn't have diet versions. I had been forced to drink sodas with sugar.

These sodas had unfamiliar flavors. Their flavors were not yet associated with calories. According to my theory, as Chapter 1 said, *a food with no flavor-calorie association will lower your set point a lot*. This made me suspect the sodas.

If my theory was wrong, to focus on soft drinks was absurd. In Paris, I surely lost weight—that's what happens when you skip meal after meal. Almost everyone thinks sugar-sweetened soft drinks cause weight *gain*. But my theory said that only *familiar* sugar-sweetened soft drinks cause weight gain (by raising the set point); *unfamiliar* ones should cause weight *loss* because they lower the set point. If my theory was right, focusing on the French soft drinks made sense.

Fructose and the Flavor–Calorie Association

When I got home, I wanted to test the idea that it was the new soft drinks that had spoiled my appetite. One test would be to drink new-flavored soft drinks and see what happened. But this would be hard to sustain: I would run out of new flavors. Another test would be to drink soft drinks with *no* flavor. With no flavor, no flavor–calorie association can form. I couldn't avoid the familiar flavor of sweetness—the drinks had to contain calories—but maybe sweetness had little effect.

The test I chose was to drink fructose-sweetened water: water with nothing but fructose. Table sugar is sucrose. Fructose is a somewhat different sugar found in honey and fruit. It looks the same as sucrose but is slightly sweeter. I used fructose instead of sucrose because fructose is digested more slowly. (Eventually I decided that the difficulties of obtaining fructose outweighed its advantages, at least for most people, and I now suggest that people use sucrose as part of the Shangri-La diet.)

I drank the fructose water "unflavored"—with nothing but fructose—to avoid forming flavor–calorie associations. Had I added lemon juice, for example, a lemon flavor–calorie association might have formed.

The fructose water caused an astonishing loss of appetite. This was clear within hours. (I started with a dose that in retrospect was much larger than necessary. With a better, lower dose, it can take longer to notice the loss of appetite.) I ate much less than usual and lost weight fast. Fructose water suppressed my appetite much more than I expected. I halved my daily intake of fructose several times over the next few weeks, yet my appetite did not return. I continued to lose weight quickly, more than two pounds per week. I simply wasn't hungry, just like in Paris. It really had been the sodas.

This was stunning. There was no precedent anywhere—not in the research literature, not in my previous self-experimentation, not in any anecdote I had ever heard—for such a small change (a few hundred calories per day) causing so much weight loss. It was much easier than any other weight-loss method I knew of. I wasn't trying to eat less (classic advice) or eat within limits (Weight Watchers) or count calories (many diets) or avoid something (Atkins, South Beach, Zone, Protein Power) or be more active (classic advice). The fructose water seemed so powerful that it appeared that I could weigh whatever I wanted. I started at 185 pounds. I decided to stop at 150 pounds, a nice round number.

I drank a small amount of fructose water every day, adjusting the quantity up and down to find a level that left me with a little bit of hunger but not a lot. Some hunger was better than none because hunger made food taste better and, of course, I still needed to eat. I ate about one meal every two days. I was never unpleasantly hungry. Sometimes I wasn't hungry enough (as in Paris). A few times I stopped the fructose water for a few days in order to increase how hungry I felt—possibly a weight-loss first.

The weight loss wasn't completely painless. It was boring to eat so little. (Slower weight loss might have solved this problem.) I often just wanted taste, not calories: I started drinking several cups of tea each day and chewing gum. I began to love super-market samples: small portions, lots of taste. I also started seeking food that was crunchy (apples, crackers, nuts, popcorn) or chewy (gum, beef jerky, dried mango). This desire for crunchy and chewy foods was new.

I reached 150 pounds in three months (see Figure 1, page 28). "Are you dying?" a colleague asked. "Don't lose any more weight," said another

Figure 1. Weight loss from fructose water. The shaded area at the bottom indicates how much fructose I drank each day.

coworker. I bought new clothes. I had my belt shortened. To stay at 150, to stop losing weight, I reduced my fructose intake. I wanted my appetite back, but I didn't want to start gaining weight. The appropriate level for me turned out to be about 3 tablespoons of fructose (150 calories) per day. Had I stopped drinking fructose altogether, I would have slowly regained the lost weight (as others do when they stop the diet). At 150 pounds, friends gently told me I looked too thin. I took their word for it and intentionally gained ten pounds.

Why did fructose water work so well? My theory had led me to this surprising discovery—so the theory surely had a lot of truth to it—but it didn't fully explain the weight loss. My theory made a prediction: *Eating calories without flavor will lower your set point.* If you consumed all of your food without any flavor, the theory said, your set point would go close to zero (almost no body fat). Something like this seems to happen in hospitals, where some patients receive all nutrition, including calories, intravenously—without any flavor, in other words. They often lose a great deal of weight and become very thin without becoming hungry. I saw a mild example of this phenomenon recently. The mother of a friend of mine spent a few days in the hospital, where she was fed intravenously. Her appetite vanished, and remained very low for several days after she left the hospital. My explanation is that due to intravenous feeding, her set point dropped quite a bit while she was in the hospital.

However, unflavored fructose water *does* have flavor: It is sweet. To explain its weight-loss potency, I had to assume that sweetness is a kind of "invisible" flavor that does not become associated with calories. This was a reasonable assumption. As a flavor becomes associated with calories, it tastes better. That's why the restaurant critic mentioned in Chapter 1 liked the taste of cilantro more and more. Sweetness, however, tastes good regardless of experience; young children naturally like sweet things. Another striking difference between sweetness and other flavors is that sweet things taste less good when you are hungry. "There is something unpleasant or aversive about sweetness when food deprivation is high," wrote Dr. Elizabeth Capaldi, a professor of psychology at the University of Florida, Gainesville, based on her research. These differences between sweetness and other flavors made it more reasonable to assume that sweetness alone did not become associated with calories (and so did not raise the set point).

Fear No Food

I stayed in the 160s—a 20-pound weight loss—without difficulty. Drinking 100 to 200 calories a day of fructose water to keep my weight in check worked well. After about two years of this, a friend pointed out that a type of olive oil, called *extra-light*, has essentially no flavor. The flavor of olive oil, if any, comes from "impurities" (molecules other than fat). Extra-virgin or virgin olive oil has a greenish color and strong taste. Extra-light olive oil (also called *pure* and *extra-light-tasting*), however, is pure fat with no flavor and no greenish tint. *Extra-light* refers to flavor, not calories. Extra-light olive oil—ELOO, I'll call it—has the same number of calories per tablespoon as other olive oils, such as extra-virgin. They all contain about 120 calories per tablespoon. My friend understood that my theory predicted that the most potent weight-loss foods provided calories without flavor. Fructose water did this because of a special wrinkle: sweetness didn't count. ELOO was another way. According to my theory, 100 calories of ELOO should have the same effect as 100 calories of fructose water.

Figure 2. Long-term effects of fructose water and extra-light olive oil.

I tested this prediction. I stopped drinking fructose water and started swallowing the same caloric amount of ELOO, about 1 tablespoon per day. I found that the prediction was right: ELOO was roughly as effective per calorie as fructose water. I stayed at the same weight. Fructose water had pushed my set point down to a certain level and kept it there; the same calorie amount of ELOO also kept it there. Figure 2 on this page, shows that I have stayed close to my chosen weight for five years.

ELOO had two advantages over fructose (and sucrose) water. First, it took less time. A day's worth could be consumed in seconds. No preparation was needed, unlike sugar water. Second, it was probably healthier than sugar water. Olive oil is a staple of the Mediterranean diet, eaten by Italians, Greeks, and Cretans, groups of people who generally enjoy long lives and have low rates of heart disease. Surveys have found that people who consume more polyunsaturated fats, including olive oil, are in better health than those who consume less. Evidence for benefits of sucrose or fructose is harder to find.

For a few years, I drank only ELOO and didn't use fructose water. Eventually I resumed drinking fructose water as well, because in small amounts it is pleasant. Then I switched from fructose water to sucrose (regular table sugar) water because sucrose is much more available. ("Free in every restaurant in America," a friend of mine likes to say.) Now I drink both: ELOO or some other flavorless oil at home, sucrose water when I'm away from home. I don't measure the amounts. If I have gained a few pounds, I drink more. If I have become too thin, I drink less.

Even when my weight was constant (in the 160s), I continued to eat much less than I had eaten when my weight was in the 180s. My metabolism had slowed down. Experiments had shown this— when you lose weight, your metabolism slows down—but their results hadn't prepared me for the size of the reduction. Before losing weight, I ate two big meals per day. After losing weight, I ate one meal per day and a few snacks. In spite of eating many fewer calories each day, I neither lost weight nor felt hungry. The time savings was wonderful. The conventional benefit of weight loss is better health: Your risk of major illnesses (diabetes, heart disease, etc.) supposedly goes down and you live longer. But it would take many years of extra life to produce the free time I save by eating one less meal per day. Because I was eating much less, I was also spending much less money on food—about half of what I had previously spent.

"Free at last," spoken softly, was how I felt. Before weight loss, I had avoided many foods I liked because I knew they would cause me to gain weight. After weight loss, with the power of fructose or sucrose or ELOO behind me, I ate whatever I wanted, in moderation. When it came to desserts, jam, pasta, bread, cookies, and other baked goods, I ate small amounts, which were plenty. Restaurant portions looked huge. Above all, I could *relax*: if something was fattening, I could simply drink more sugar water the next day. Not only could I eat anything, I could also eat nothing—skip any meal—and feel fine. On a long flight, for example, if I didn't like the airplane food, I simply didn't eat it. Because I ate much less, I was happy to pay much more per meal. Food became less a necessity and more a treat. I was careful to get good nutrition (fruits, vegetables, whole grains, vitamins and minerals) every day.

My Eureka Moment

According to *New Yorker* writer Malcolm Gladwell, diet books "have an unspoken set of narrative rules and conventions," which include "the Eureka

Moment, when the author explains how he stumbled on the radical truth that inspired his diet." I too had a Eureka Moment, but it was not the sugar-water discovery.

It happened long before that: when I discovered that the weight-loss advice I had been giving my students actually worked. One conclusion in my lecture on weight control was that *the better food tastes, the more fattening it is*. What makes food taste good? Well, processing helps. Much of what we do to food improves the taste. This suggested that less-processed food—food closer to its natural state—would be less good tasting and therefore less fattening. I tested this prediction. I ate less-processed food: oranges instead of orange juice, brown rice instead of white rice or pasta, simple home-cooked food instead of take-out or deli food. I stopped eating baked goods, including bread. For the first few days, the new food seemed bland and dull. Within a week, however, I came to enjoy it and found my former food unappetizing.

As mentioned earlier, it worked. I lost ten pounds in eight weeks (see Figure 3, page 35). Apart from the modest difficulty involved in changing what I ate, it was effortless. For a while I felt less hungry than usual, so I ate less than usual and thereby lost weight. I never regained the lost weight. I never missed the food I stopped eating. Even now, fifteen years later, I still dislike orange juice and scones. The consensus among weight-loss experts has been that it is nearly impossible to lose weight

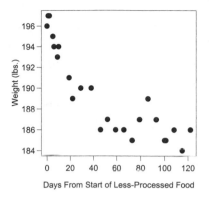

Figure 3. Weight loss when I started eating less-processed food—oranges instead of orange juice, for example.

and keep it off. "Weight loss is not for the faint-hearted," said Dr. Thomas Wadden, director of the Weight and Eating Disorders Program at the University of Pennsylvania, in 2005. But I had lost weight easily.

The "radical truth" that inspired my diet was not that eating less-processed food caused me to lose weight. That was just an interesting truth. The radical truth was how easy it had been to learn that interesting truth. I could not explain why my dietary change had caused weight loss. But I realized *I might be able to find out by studying myself.* In a world where a typical weight-loss study costs hundreds of thousands of dollars, takes several years, and is done by a team of scientists who have devoted their professional lives to the subject, to believe that someone like me—basically ignorant, with no credentials in physiology or nutrition—

could learn something important at no cost in a few months *was* radical. Self-experimentation has a long history in medicine, but it has almost always been used to show rather than to find. For example, Barry Marshall, winner of the 2005 Nobel Prize in Medicine, used his own body to show the truth of an idea about ulcers. The self-experimentation came long after the idea. My notion was that self-experimentation could *give* me ideas.

That is what happened. My weight control theory was initially inspired by some rat experiments done by Israel Ramirez (see Appendix). But I came to believe the theory because it helped me find new ways of losing weight. When I lost my appetite in Paris, I believed my theory strongly enough to test the hypothesis that it suggested: that my loss of appetite was due to drinking sodas with unfamiliar flavors. And that hypothesis—which would strike most people, including most obesity researchers, as absurd—turned out to be correct.

⤳ Two Turkeys

SARAH's problem with her weight began when she was young. "When I was nine, I weighed 109," she said. "That's a lot." Growing up, she always weighed more than she wanted to.

In her forties, she tried Weight Watchers, which worked for a while. She lost twenty-five pounds, ultimately reaching her goal weight of 145—a good weight for her height of five foot seven. Eventually, however, she stopped following the plan. Over the next twenty years, she gained fifty pounds, reaching 195 pounds.

Sarah began the Shangri-La diet (the early, fructose-water version) in 2001 when she was sixty-one. Over eight months, she lost forty pounds and stayed at the lower weight (see Figure 4, page 38). During this time, she continued to eat three meals a day. She also continued her exercise routine (elliptical trainer or stationary bike for thirty to forty minutes three times a week). She didn't change what she ate; she just ate less of it. She played a little game with herself. She would look at the food in front of her and think, *How little can I eat and still feel satisfied?* After she started drinking fructose water, the answer was about half the amount of food she usually ate. She loved the lack of restrictions on what she could eat. "If I felt like having pizza, I'd just eat one piece—and I was satisfied

Figure 4. Sarah's weight over time. The open circles show her weight before starting the diet. The shaded area shows how much fructose she drank each day. The wider gaps indicate vacations; the thin gaps indicate weekends. Starting around day 300, she drank the sugar water only during the week.

with that." Rather than following rigid rules about how much she could eat, as Weight Watchers had required, she could simply eat enough to feel satisfied.

Sarah had no problem with hunger while she was drinking fructose water. Instead, as she ate much less due to being less hungry, food became "an event—not something you gobble down or sneak." She started drinking fructose water in September; by Christmas, she had lost twenty pounds. Taking a Christmas turkey out of the refrigerator, she realized, "I had lost a real burden"— the weight of a large turkey. She and her friends invented a weight-loss unit called the *turkey*: 1 turkey = 20 lbs. Eventually she lost two turkeys. When she reached her chosen weight, she gradually cut back the fructose so that she wouldn't lose any more.

Sarah went from a size eighteen to a size twelve. She was delighted that she no longer had to shop in plus-sized clothing stores. "After I lost weight, I could walk into an ordinary store, and the clothes would actually fit me. That was very nice." Also very nice were the improvements in her health. Her blood pressure went from 140/80 (borderline high) to 110/70 (normal). "My kids were in awe about what I had accomplished. It made me feel great that they were proud of me. It's certainly nice to have people compliment me on my appearance, but it's not as important as my sense of achievement. I felt I had a huge success at a battle I had been fighting my whole life."

3

A NEW THEORY OF WEIGHT CONTROL

THIS CHAPTER explains the theory behind the diet. The theory doesn't merely explain why the diet works; it actually helped me discover it. After calorielab.com posted a long and skeptical account of this diet, someone commented, "I have been using the Shangri-La diet now for almost a month, and it works beautifully. . . . Who cares why?" Well, yes, not everyone cares. You don't need to understand the theory to do well with the diet. But I think some readers will want to. Maybe it will help *you* discover new ways of losing weight.

The theory consists of several interlocking ideas, which I will explain one by one.

Idea 1. Your weight is regulated by a system with a set point.

As Chapter 1, "Why a Calorie Is Not a Calorie," discussed, your body's weight-control system resembles a thermostat-controlled heating system. Just as a thermostat-controlled heating system has a set-point temperature that it tries to maintain, your body's weight-control system has a set-point *weight* that it tries to maintain. The Appendix, "The Science Behind the Theory Behind the Diet," describes some of the evidence for this idea.

The name *set point* may be confusing because the set point is *not* fixed or "set"; it may help to remember that the temperature to which a thermostat is set is not fixed either. *Set point* is just one of those terms whose meaning is quite different from the sum of its parts.

Idea 2. When your actual weight falls below your set point, your system makes you more hungry and increases how much food it takes to make you feel full.

When a thermostat detects that the room temperature is lower than the set point, it turns on the heat to warm up the room. Turning on the heat pushes the temperature back up toward the set point. When the temperature reaches the set point, the heat is turned off. When your body-weight regulatory system detects that you have less fat on your body than your set point, it makes you more hungry than usual between meals and increases how much food you need to eat to feel full. (There are other changes too, but these are the most obvious.) These changes cause you to eat more than usual and gain weight—pushing your weight back up toward your set point. As your weight gets closer to your set point, your hunger goes down.

Idea 3. Between meals, your set point goes down.

When you are not eating, your set point slowly goes down. The rate of decline varies widely (see Idea 4), but a very rough estimate is a half pound per day. (When you don't eat, your weight goes down too, of course, as you burn fat. Your weight goes down faster than your set point. That is why not eating causes hunger—and why diets that deprive you of food don't work.)

Idea 4. The higher your set point, the faster it goes down between meals.

If your set point is very high (you are obese), it may decrease between meals at the rate of one pound per day. If your set point is quite low (you are thin), it will decrease much more slowly—perhaps a quarter pound per day.

Idea 5. Eating flavors that are associated with calories raises your set point.

When you eat something with a calorie-associated flavor, your set point goes up. Any familiar food with calories (apple, bread, salmon) will do this.

Ideas 3 and 5 together imply that your set point is always going up and down: up at a meal (Idea 5), down between meals (Idea 3), up at a meal, down, etc. Figure 5 below shows this oscillation.

Your set point will stay roughly the same—going up and down around the same value—only if the amount that food raises your set point *at* meals equals the amount that your set point goes down *between* meals. The chances are very good that right now this is true: The food you eat raises your set point by the same amount that it declines between meals. This keeps your set point stable—and therefore keeps your weight stable. (Your weight is always close to your set point.) The Shangri-La diet causes weight loss because it reduces how much your food increases your set point each day—you get the same number of calories but your set point goes up less. The result is that your current set point—and therefore your current weight—become unsustainable. Your set point will slowly fall until increase and decrease are back in balance.

For example, suppose your food increases your set point by 1 pound per day and your set point decreases between meals by 1 pound per day. This is a stable situation: Your set point will go up and

Figure 5. The effect of food on your set point.

down around the same value, day after day after day. January, February, March—your weight stays the same. On April 1 you change your diet so that your set point goes up only 0.8 pound per day. This is *not* a stable situation. Your set point goes down between meals more than it goes up at meals. The level around which your set point oscillates will gradually decrease—by 0.2 pound per day. Because this level is decreasing, you will lose weight. April, May, June, you lose weight. You will lose weight until you reach a weight at which your set point goes down only 0.8 pound per day between meals instead of 1 pound per day.

Idea 6. The stronger a food's flavor–calorie association, the more your set point will go up when you eat it.

The strength of the flavor-calorie association matters: Flavors strongly associated with calories raise your set point more than flavors weakly associated with calories. Below, in "Applying the Theory to Everyday Foods," page 46, I will explain what makes a flavor-calorie association strong or weak.

You can get some sense of how strongly a flavor is associated with calories. A flavor not associated with calories tastes a bit flat and/or strange, or even unpleasant. As the flavor-calorie association becomes stronger, the flavor doesn't exactly change, but it becomes pleasant and familiar. You can experience this for yourself by drinking an unfamiliar tea. Add sugar to the tea (for calories). The first cup will taste mildly pleasant because of the sweetness of the sugar. If you have one cup of tea with sugar per day, subsequent cups will taste better and better as the flavor of the tea becomes associated with the calories in the sugar. If, on the other hand, you add a noncaloric sweetener (such as Splenda) to the tea, subsequent cups will *not* taste better and better. The tea's flavor will not become associated with calories because the drink has no calories.

You probably have several favorite foods that taste very good to you due to very strong flavor-calorie associations. These will always be foods that you have eaten many times. A chocolate-covered doughnut? A hot dog with a certain type of mustard? A glass of Scotch? If there are foods you crave, foods that bring great pleasure, foods you can't go a day without eating (if you are Pepsiholic, for instance), food you would drive thirty minutes for—those are examples. Eating these foods causes your set point to go up—more so than when you eat foods that aren't as familiar or flavorful.

At the low end of the strength-of-association scale are flavors not associated with calories. This is where every flavor begins. The very first time you taste any flavor, it has no association with calories. By the time you are old enough to read this book, however, almost everything you eat tastes at least somewhat familiar. The average person encounters completely unfamiliar flavors when being adventurous (going to an unusual ethnic restaurant, making a recipe with unusual ingredients or spice combinations) or when in a foreign country. I shop in many ethnic food stores, where I buy packaged foods with unfamiliar flavors—my version of armchair tourism. Eating unfamiliar foods does not raise your set point, so these foods offer a rare opportunity to fly under the radar of your body's weight-regulating system and eat without raising your set point.

Applying the Theory to Everyday Foods

How can we use this theory to figure out what to eat to lose weight? We need to figure out which foods when eaten many times have strong flavor-calorie associations and which have weak associations.

One hundred years of research on Pavlovian conditioning comes to our rescue here. This research has established two rules that have been found to apply to all examples of Pavlovian conditioning.

First, *the weaker the signal, the weaker the association*. If Pavlov used a bell that the dogs could barely hear, it would produce less salivation than a bell the dogs could hear clearly.

Applied to flavor-calorie learning, this means that *the weaker a food's flavor, the weaker its flavor-calorie association*. If you reduce the amount of flavor in your food, the flavor-calorie associations will become weaker. When I started eating large amounts of a relatively bland food (sushi) I did in fact lose weight. I later discovered that sugar water and extra-light olive oil—both of which have no flavor—worked even better.

Second, *the more delayed the outcome, the weaker the association.* In Pavlov's experiments, the bell was the signal and the food was the outcome. The food was given at the same time the bell was turned off. Had the food been given many minutes after the bell was turned off, the dog would not have associated them at all.

Applied to flavor-calorie learning, this means *the slower a food is digested, the weaker its flavor-calorie association.* When a food is digested more slowly, the calories in that food are detected more slowly. Thus there is more of a gap between the signal (flavor) and the outcome (calories). I believe this is why low-carb and good-carb diets work: They replace foods that are digested quickly, such as bread, with foods that are digested slowly, such as vegetables. The foods that are digested more slowly have weaker flavor-calorie associations. They raise your set point less.

A Stone Age Grain Elevator

It's no great puzzle why our weight-regulation system works this way. It is a system designed to stock up on energy (calories)—that is, make us fatter—when food is plentiful and to reduce the amount of energy stored—make us thinner—when food is scarce. This is the way any sensible commodity storage system works. I stock up on paper towels when they are cheap and use what I have stored when they are expensive. Grain elevators store grain when it is cheap. The stored grain is sold when it is more expensive.

The system I've described uses the flavor of foods to determine whether food is plentiful or scarce. In Stone Age times of plenty, food tasted better. In the Stone Age, when food was plentiful the best-tasting foods—those with the strongest flavor-calorie associations—were more likely to be eaten than when food was scarce.

In the Stone Age, this system made us fat, or at least fatter, during "fat years," as protection against "lean years" to come. But nowadays, the lean years never come, and our once-precious fat does more harm than good.

Why Believe It?

No one believes a theory but the theorist, the saying goes. It's not entirely true. Two sorts of findings are especially persuasive. First, confirmation of a surprising prediction. A famous example is the return of Halley's Comet at the predicted time—very convincing evidence for the theory that comets orbit the sun. One surprising prediction of this weight-control theory that has been confirmed is that extra-light olive oil will cause weight loss. The usual idea has been that consuming fat causes weight gain. Second, repeated usefulness. When a theory is useful again and again, skepticism melts away. This theory led me to try a low glycemic index diet. That worked: I lost weight. It led me to eat lots of sushi. That worked. It led me to drink sugar water. That worked extremely well. It led me to drink extra-light olive oil. That worked extremely well too.

For more about the theory, see my paper "What makes food fattening? A Pavlovian theory of weight control" at www.sethroberts.net/articles/whatmakesfoodfattening.pdf.

⤳ Food Falls on
the Floor

WHEN Michael was forty-eight, he weighed 254 pounds. He is six feet tall. He had been heavy since grade school. "I was a short, fat kid with a crew cut," he told me. Quite apart from health issues— his knees hurt, for one thing—his weight was a problem because it caused people to treat him poorly. "Society establishes that since you are fat, you have no worth," he said.

His eyes lit up when he heard from a coworker that I had lost weight simply by drinking fructose water. *I can do that,* he thought. "It was like someone throwing me a life preserver. I was going to be rescued from being a lot heavier than I wanted to be. I'd been waiting a long time for this." Michael had wanted to lose weight for a long time, but he didn't want to eat special food. That meant no Atkins, no Jenny Craig. He passed Weight Watchers on his way to work, but "the idea of going in there and being the only man in a room full of women didn't appeal to me."

He started drinking six tablespoons of fructose (mixed into one quart of water) each day. On most days, he ate just one meal, at lunchtime: about three ounces of protein (tofu, chicken, or fish) plus a big salad. No breakfast, no snacks, no dinner. When he and his wife had a meal away from home—at his parents' house, for instance—he ate whatever was served, including dessert, but found that he ate less than he had previously.

Michael's wife loved that he was losing weight but hated eating dinner alone on the nights they were home. On the other hand, they spent time together in a new way. Most evenings, they took a fast-paced forty-five-minute walk together, up and down hills.

Soon after Michael started drinking fructose water, it was clear it was working. He lost weight steadily. After he had lost twenty pounds, the mutual friend who had told him about my fructose-water plan wrote to me: "Every day he thanks me. Says he's going to name all his children after me if he ever has any." He lost weight steadily (see Figure 6, page 52). Eleven months after starting the fructose regimen, he weighed 173 pounds, a loss of eighty pounds. In fact, he weighed less than his maximum weight during high school. He usually wore black. A coworker joked that he had gone from Orson Welles to Johnny Cash.

Some of the benefits of weight loss were physical. When Michael was heavy, he sometimes snored loudly. After his weight loss, the snoring stopped. His knee pain went away. Other changes were social. His office used to be called *the crying room*, he told me, because some of his female coworkers would routinely come to talk to him about their guy problems. When he lost the weight, they stopped telling him their sad stories. "If you're heavier,

Figure 6. Michael's weight over time. The shaded area shows how much fructose he drank each day. The open circles show his weight before starting the diet.

you're thought of as just a buddy. Fat guys aren't really considered men," he said. Friendly sexual banter from his female coworkers slowed and stopped as he went from 250 to 170. "At 250, I could never take it the wrong way, they figured. It's inconceivable that what they are saying to you could ever happen," Michael said. "At 170, they think: Maybe he'll think I'm coming on to him instead of teasing him."

Michael's new physique also elicited a new response from a particularly nasty coworker. When he was heavy, Michael said, "whenever this woman talked to me her attitude toward me was, like, *you lowly piece of* ———. When I weighed 173, she treated me the same way she treated everyone else." After losing all that weight, Michael said, strangers smiled at him more. I repeated this to one of Michael's coworkers. "*He* smiles more," she said.

Someone else at work had also lost a lot of weight. One day Michael told him, "The best thing about being thin is that food falls on the floor" (instead of on your shirt). They laughed. It was a joke not everyone understood, Michael told me.

4

HOW TO DO THE SHANGRI-LA DIET

Secretly, I suspected the answer to weight issues
would be something ridiculously simple,
but this is almost too much to hope for.

—*Starkville Daily News*

It appealed to my essential laziness.

—A BLOGGER'S REASON FOR TRYING
THE SHANGRI-LA DIET

THE SHANGRI-LA diet is the most flexible weight-loss plan yet devised. No forbidden foods, no restricted foods, no calorie counting, no meal plans, no recipes, and, above all, no deprivation. No subtraction, just addition. Just follow the flexible basic framework and choose among the many possibilities it allows.

The Big Picture

The big picture of the Shangri-La diet is very simple. There are only two rules:

Rule 1. Take 100 to 400 calories of sugar water and/or flavorless edible oil daily.

The total number of calories is what matters. One hundred calories of sugar water will have the same effect as 100 calories of flavorless oil. The more calories you consume this way, the more weight you will lose—as odd as that may sound. Flavorless edible oils include extra-light olive oil (ELOO), safflower oil, and canola oil, but any flavorless oil will do.

I recommend starting with both sugar water *and* flavorless oil. Two small amounts (for example, 50 calories of sugar water and 150 calories of flavorless oil) are likely to be better digested than one larger amount (200 calories of only flavorless oil).

How much you should take depends on how much weight you want to lose. Consult the table on page 56 to choose a starting amount. The sugar amounts in the table are how much sugar you dissolve in water—the amount of water is up to you, as I'll explain a little later in this chapter. After a few weeks or a month you will probably adjust the values up or down to lose weight faster or slower. Don't try to lose more than two pounds per week. That's generally considered a healthy rate of weight loss.

Rule 2. Take the sugar water and/or oil well before or well after meals—at least an hour away.

For example, if you expect to eat lunch from noon to 1 p.m., take the sugar water or oil by 11 a.m. or

How Much Sugar and Oil to Take

IF YOU WANT TO LOSE . . .	SUGAR IN WATER	SUGAR CALORIES	OIL	OIL CALORIES	TOTAL CALORIES
Less than 20 lbs.	1 Tbsp./day	45	1 Tbsp./day	120	165
20–40 lbs.	2 Tbsp./day	90	2 Tbsp./day	240	330
More than 40 lbs.	3 Tbsp./day	135	2 Tbsp./day	240	375

after 2 p.m. Beyond the basic idea of taking the sugar water or oil at least an hour away from a meal (and all other food), however, the time of day doesn't matter. If you take both sugar and oil, you can take them at the same time or at different times. The time of day doesn't matter because the sugar water and oil are not short-acting appetite suppressants that reduce appetite for a few hours. Their effects last a long time.

Unless the daily amount you plan to take is small (one tablespoon per day or less), divide it into at least two portions that you take at different times. What works well for many people is to take the first portion between breakfast and lunch and the second after dinner. The more slowly you take the oil and sugar water, the more easily your body will digest them.

What about the rest of what you eat? *Adding the sugar water and oil are the only changes you need to make in your diet.* You don't have to consciously eat less of anything or watch what you eat. You will be a lot less hungry and you will find that you eat less and feel full faster. The overall result will be that you take in fewer calories and lose weight without making a deliberate effort to choose lower-calorie foods or eat less. A very nice feature of this diet is that it will help you make better dietary choices because it will reduce or eliminate your cravings for junk foods. Most diets make life harder; this one makes life easier. See "In Shangri-La," pages 90–97, for many examples.

Preparing the Sugar Water

You can make the sugar water with sucrose (ordinary sugar) or fructose (fruit sugar). They are equally effective. Keep in mind:

- The sugar water *must* be unflavored. The Shangri-La diet works because it gives you calories without flavor. (Sweetness does not count as a flavor.) This is why drinking sugar-sweetened soft drinks, such as Coke, does not work. (It would be the best-kept secret in world history if drinking Coke caused weight loss.) *Don't add anything to the sugar water*—not even lemon juice, for example.

- The sugar water *must* have calories. Water sweetened with sucralose (Splenda), aspartame

(NutraSweet, Equal), saccharin (Sweet'n Low), or stevia will not work. One Shangri-La dieter started with sugar water, lost some weight, and thought it was the sweet taste of the water that made the difference. She switched to water sweetened with Splenda. About a week later, her appetite began to return and she started to regain the lost weight.

Ordinary white table sugar, or sucrose, is the easiest and cheapest sugar to use. To avoid flavor, you must use only white sugar, not brown sugar, raw sugar, or molasses. In five-pound bags, 100 calories of sucrose costs three cents. I like my sugar water hot, like tea, but that's just a personal preference. (It is a good idea to drink the sugar water slowly, and hot water will force you to do this.) You can drink it at any temperature you like. If you prefer it cool or cold, try using confectioners' sugar (six cents for 100 calories), which is extra-fine powdered sugar. It dissolves in cold water more quickly than table sugar.

Fructose is a natural sugar found in honey, fruit, and soft drinks sweetened with high-fructose corn syrup. If you drink any sort of mass-produced soft drink (soda, energy drinks, sports drinks, and the like), you're already consuming a lot of fructose, because these drinks are sweetened with high-fructose corn syrup, not sucrose. Granular fructose that you can stir into water can be a little hard to find. It is sold in bulk at Whole Foods and similar stores, at about a dollar per pound, or six cents per 100 calories. At health food stores, it may cost much more.

Should you use sucrose or fructose?

I now use sucrose. However, I discovered the powerful weight-loss effects of sugar water using fructose. I chose fructose rather than sucrose to avoid large changes in my blood sugar level. Fructose has a much lower glycemic index than sucrose, which indicates that it has less effect on your blood sugar. Another reason I chose fructose instead of sucrose is that rat experiments had found that it is relatively hard to produce flavor-calorie associations when fructose is the source of the calories.

Now and then people tell me that fructose gave them headaches or indigestion, perhaps because it was unfamiliar to their digestive systems and not digested well. Rather than wastefully produce all possible digestive enzymes all the time, your body makes only those that it actually needs. When a food requiring new digestive enzymes is eaten, your body starts making more of those enzymes. If any of the foods you eat for this diet (the sugar water and/or the oil) are new to you, you should start with small amounts (one tablespoon or less) for the first few days.

Because sucrose is much more convenient than fructose, and I found it equally effective, I now prefer it. If you are worried about your blood sugar level, you might prefer fructose or might want to take only the oil instead.

Whichever sugar you choose, *you should sip the sugar water slowly.* This will minimize the burden on your pancreas, which produces insulin, and minimize changes in your blood sugar. One blogger reported, "About an hour after I drank the sugar water [three tablespoons in a large glass of water] I got very sleepy." This was probably due to drinking the sugar water too quickly. As the sugar is digested in your stomach and converted to glucose (blood sugar), your blood sugar level (the concentration of glucose in your blood) goes up. When your blood sugar goes up, your body makes insulin in order to lower it. If too much insulin is made in response to the sugar water, as can happen with some people, your blood sugar then goes too low and you may become sleepy or start to feel tired and a little shaky. If I eat a bread roll on an empty stomach (somehow I always eat it quickly), I become sleepy a half hour later, no doubt due to low blood sugar. (Bread has a high glycemic index.) If you drink the sugar water slowly, however, it will have the same effect on your blood sugar level as eating a piece of fruit. Sip the sugar water slowly over thirty minutes or more rather than swallowing it all at once.

Another reason to sip the sugar water slowly is to avoid a yeast infection. Women who are prone to yeast infections should either dilute the sugar a great deal or drink the oil instead.

How much water should I use?

The amount of water in which you dissolve the sugar will not affect the power of the sugar to reduce your weight. You can suck on sugar cubes and get the same effect. However, *the more slowly you consume the sugar, the better*. Mix the sugar with as much water as you can easily drink in thirty minutes or so. This will slow down how quickly you ingest it.

The typical amount of water most Shangri-La dieters use is one cup of water per tablespoon of sugar. (Bear in mind that one tablespoon of sugar is the equivalent of three teaspoons or three to four packets of sugar.) That amount might be too sweet for your taste, however, or not sweet enough. Adjust

HOW MUCH WATER SHOULD I USE?

AMOUNT OF SUGAR	SWEETNESS		
	HIGH	AVERAGE	LOW
1 Tbsp.	6 oz./200 ml	1 cup/250 ml	12 oz./350 ml
2 Tbsp.	1.5 cups/350 ml	2 cups/500 ml	3 cups/750 ml
3 Tbsp.	2.2 cups/500 ml	3 cups/750 ml	4.5 cups/1 liter
4 Tbsp.	3 cups/750 ml	4 cups/1 liter	6 cups/1.5 liters

the amount of water to find a level of sweetness you like. The table on page 61 gives some possibilities.

Flavorless Oils

For the edible oil option to work, the oil must have little or no flavor. When I began using oil, for two years I used extra-light olive oil (the label may read *extra-light-tasting* or *extra-light in taste*). Extra-light olive oil (ELOO) has the same number of calories per ounce as extra-virgin olive oil (EVOO). The term *light* refers to its taste and appearance. ELOO is flavorless and more transparent than EVOO, which is greenish. More recently, I have used canola oil and safflower oil as well. Both are nearly flavorless. If the oil has a strong flavor, the flavor will become associated with calories; then the oil will begin to raise your set point, and its appetite-reducing effect will be lost. One Shangri-La dieter wrote, "I would gulp a spoonful and I could almost feel something primal going yeah, gimme more of

FLAVORLESS OILS

TYPE	COST PER 100 CALORIES	OTHER BENEFITS
Canola	2 cents	Good source of omega-3 fatty acids
Safflower	6 cents	High in polyunsaturated fat
Extra-light olive oil	15 cents	Part of Mediterranean diet

DISGUSTOLOGY: THE PROBLEM WITH OIL

Two years ago I visited Xiaochi Jie (Snack Street) in Beijing, China. It was lined with stalls selling exotic foods: grasshoppers, bees, silkworm grubs, starfish, goat testicles, and sparrows, to name a few. My reaction, unfortunately, was: *No way!* I think of myself as an adventurous eater, but I did not try even one of them. It was curious that I had such a strong aversion to things I knew nothing about. I don't have a strong aversion to books I haven't read, or films I haven't seen, or music I haven't heard. Just certain foods I've never tasted.

Billions of people drink sugar water every day. Few people drink edible oils regularly. I find ELOO, canola oil, and many other oils, such as safflower oil, easy to swallow in single-tablespoon amounts. The very first time I drank ELOO I was apprehensive, but after that it was easy. Now the experience is neutral: neither pleasant nor unpleasant. Some people, however, find the very thought of drinking oil off-putting—like my reaction to the thought of eating bees.

To learn more about this reaction, I spoke with Paul Rozin, a professor of psychology at the University of Pennsylvania, who has studied disgust for more than twenty years. One of his conclusions is that disgust is usually learned from others. It transmits cultural values. "Our subjects have told us that racists, child abusers, hypocrites, Republicans and liberals are all disgusting," he has written. In the case of oils, "it has always puzzled me," he said, "that people never drink oils, especially nicely flavored oils, like sesame and olive. I think it could easily be otherwise."

Rozin added: "I doubt that infants are averse to eating oil; they like eating fatty things." Several people have told me that when they were children their mothers gave them castor oil. Now when they drink olive oil to lose weight, they find it comforting. This suggests that early experience matters; maybe while I was growing up, grasshoppers, bees, and so on, came to be labeled *don't eat* in my mind.

If disgust is learned, it can be unlearned. If the Shangri-La diet becomes popular, and many people drink ELOO regularly, the idea that drinking oil is disgusting may be replaced by the idea that it is healthy. Rozin also pointed out that people are quite poor at predicting how they will react to something after repeated exposures. They badly underestimate how much they will get used to it, he said. In the case of oils, this means that what you find disgusting now will become acceptable more quickly than you probably think. The experience of one Shangri-La dieter bears this out. "When I began [drinking olive oil]," she told me, "it was really gross. Now it's fine. It's unpleasant, but not a big deal. A lot less gross. Now that I know what to expect, it's not as bad as I thought it would be." She holds the tablespoon really close, drinks it fast, and takes a big swig of water afterward to wash the oily feel out of her mouth.

dat. So even though it was light-tasting, maybe my body finally figured out it was a rich food source." If you start to like the taste of the oil, something is wrong. Change oils.

An unexpected benefit, several people have told

me, is that ELOO made their skin softer. Someone else said that canola oil had this effect. Other oils would probably do the same.

If ELOO or any other oil doesn't suppress your appetite within a few days, don't give up. You may not yet be digesting it properly. It may take several days of exposure for your digestive system to make enough of the enzymes you need to digest an unfamiliar food.

Sugar or Oil?

Both work. Many people strongly prefer one or the other. For example, people who are diabetic will obviously prefer oil. People who are on a low-carb diet will prefer oil. People who are on a low-fat diet will prefer sugar water. In any case, choose what works best for you.

About half the Shangri-La dieters I encounter prefer sugar water, about half prefer oil. I prefer oil. At home, it is much faster and easier than sugar water, which requires mixing and sipping. Away from home, however, sugar water is much easier than oil. At a café, hot sugar water is convenient, tasty, pleasantly warm on a cold day, and a good excuse for a break. I believe that small daily amounts of sugar water, consumed slowly, carry little or no health risk, but that large daily amounts of sugar water, drunk quickly, may be damaging because of the high blood sugar levels they repeatedly cause.

Unflavored sugar water and commercial soft drinks, such as Coke and Pepsi, differ by only a tiny amount, in the sense that the flavorings in Coke or Pepsi are a very small fraction of their weight (0.001 percent?). Yet this tiny difference in ingredients has a huge effect on how we respond to them. The difference emphasized in this book is that you can drink unflavored sugar water to lose weight; of course, you can't drink Coke or Pepsi to do so. Another interesting difference is that unflavored sugar water, unlike commercial soft drinks, never becomes addictive.

Dr. William Jacobs is a professor of psychiatry at the University of Florida's College of Medicine, where he specializes in addiction medicine, and has directed the department's Overeating and Eating Disorders Clinic. He has never seen anyone addicted to unflavored sugar water, but he *has* seen hundreds of people addicted to commercial soft drinks, such as Coke, Pepsi, and Mountain Dew. A typical soft drink addict drinks two or three liters per day, said Jacobs. I believe that Coke, Pepsi, and the like can become addictive because they can produce very strong flavor-calorie associations. A food with a very strong flavor-calorie association tastes very good, which is why it is addictive; such food raises the set point a great deal, which is why soft drink addicts end up at an overeating (obesity) clinic. Sugar water, without flavor, has no flavor-calorie association. Sweetness makes it pleasant to drink; but it never becomes addictive because without flavor there can be no very strong flavor-calorie association.

All plants contain sugar. They use it to transport energy, just as our bodies do. Fruits contain plenty of sugar—a banana has the equivalent of about two tablespoons of sucrose. Unlike the sugar in most fruits, however, the sugar in sugar water is digested quickly and can cause a sharp increase in your blood sugar level. It is only this blood sugar spike that is "unnatural" and possibly damaging. If you drink sugar water slowly, there will be no spike.

Results from the Nurses' Health Study, which has followed the health of over one hundred thousand women for almost thirty years, suggest that there indeed is reason to be concerned about sharp rises in blood sugar that happen day after day for years. Researchers found that women who drank at least one sugar-sweetened drink per day had a 40 percent higher risk of Type 2 diabetes than women who drank less than one per month. The risk was corrected for weight, meaning that the increased risk was not due to a weight difference between the two groups of women. These results are more evidence that sugar water should be consumed slowly, around thirty minutes per serving.

Sugar should not be demonized, but it is true that sugar water is empty calories in a way that olive oil, safflower oil, and canola oil are not. Study after study has found benefits from consuming mono- or polyunsaturated fats, the so-called good fats. Olive oil, canola oil, and safflower oil are all good sources of good fats. The nutrition guide *Eat, Drink, and Be Healthy* (2001), by Walter C. Willett, has an excellent discussion of their benefits. "Eating more good fats—and staying away from the bad ones—is second only to weight control on the list of healthy nutritional strategies," Willett writes. He is one of the leaders of the Nurses' Health Study, and bases his recommendation on years of analyzing data from the study.

A famous clinical trial called the Lyon Diet Heart Study, which began in 1988 and ran for five years, measured the effect of two different diets on people who had already had one heart attack. Half of the subjects were told to follow a low-fat diet recommended by the American Heart Association; the other half were told to follow a Mediterranean diet that included plenty of olive oil and canola oil. Those who ate the Mediterranean diet had half as many deaths from all causes over the next four years as those who ate the low-fat diet—a huge difference. Heart attack deaths in the Mediterranean group went down by two-thirds. The reduction in heart attacks became apparent within months of starting the diet. Drinking olive oil will probably have more benefits than just weight loss.

How Much?

People who have followed the Shangri-La diet have had excellent results when the total amount of sugar water and/or oil was no more than 400 calories per day. Even people who have consumed much less—only 200 calories total—notice results.

Whatever amount you choose—100, 200, or 400 calories per day—you should lose weight steadily, allowing for plateaus now and then, for several months. Eventually you will stop losing weight and may regain a small portion of the lost weight. This is normal. *It does not mean that the sugar water and/or oil have stopped working.* I call this *overshoot*: Your weight goes below the level that you will be able to sustain with the amounts of sugar and/or oil you are taking.

To take much more than 400 calories per day of sugar water and/or oil for a long period of time (months) is to venture into unknown territory. Consuming a great deal of any one or two foods is usually a bad idea in terms of overall nutrition. Rather than increasing your intake above 400 calories of sugar water and/or oil per day, I suggest supplementing the diet with one or more of the weight-loss methods explained in Chapter 6, "Extra Credit: Six More Ways to Lose Weight."

The One-Hour Rule

The second rule is to take the sugar water or oil at least one hour away from a meal. If you take the sugar water or oil at a meal, they will simply act as added calories, strengthening the flavor-calorie associations of whatever you are eating. That's the opposite of what you want to do.

Many experiments with rats have found that adding sugar water to the diet causes weight gain.

I believe this is because the sugar water is available at the same time as the rest of the food. The same may be true of taking oil with a meal. I spoke to a woman who lost weight while swallowing fish oil capsules between meals (for health reasons—she was doing the Shangri-La diet by accident) but gained weight when she began swallowing them at the same time as meals.

How far from meals should the sugar or oil be? I chose the value of one hour—in other words, the sugar or oil should be taken at least one hour away from meals—based on two sets of rat experiments. One set found that a flavor-calorie association was learned even when there was a thirty-minute gap between eating the flavor source and eating the calorie source. The other set found that a one-hour interval between flavor and calorie source was enough to prevent a flavor-calorie association from being learned.

Results tend to be better when people take the sugar or oil one hour after a meal rather than one hour before a meal. After taking the sugar or oil, you must wait an hour before eating something (water doesn't count). This is easier to do after a meal, when you're full, than before a meal, when you're probably hungry.

If you have trouble remembering to take the sugar or oil, it may help to attach it to something you already do, something that is already part of your daily routine. One person takes the sugar water first thing in the morning when he gets up and last thing in the evening before he goes to bed. You might attach it to walking the dog, leaving for work, midmorning break at the office, or coming home from work.

Don't wait for hunger pangs. One person using sugar water compared two ways of doing it: waiting until she got hungry to drink it; and drinking it an hour after breakfast and an hour after lunch. It worked much better to drink it an hour after breakfast and lunch. Someone else had a similar experience. It worked better to drink the sugar water at regular intervals than to wait until he felt hungry to drink it.

Your Real Food

The rest of what you eat, in addition to the sugar water and/or oil, can be anything you want. However, an unhealthy diet is still an unhealthy diet. While you're losing weight, you'll be eating relatively small amounts of "real food"—that is, meals and snacks—because you simply won't be hungry enough to eat large portions. Make those small amounts as nutritious and healthy as possible. You may also want to take a multivitamin supplement as insurance to be sure you're getting adequate amounts of essential nutrients.

This finger-wagging tone doesn't do justice to how people actually feel about their food while on the Shangri-La diet. "I ate *pesto* yesterday (home-made) with lots of olive oil and nuts. . . . Pesto never would have been allowed on a conventional plan. Hooray!" (Homemade food is always a good idea. See Method 2 in Chapter 6, "Extra Credit: Six More Ways to Lose Weight," page 101.)

When you are losing weight, you will of course be eating less than usual because you will be a lot less hungry. My solution was to eat only one normal-sized meal per day. Sometimes lunch, sometimes dinner—it depended on who I was eating with. Some people who have done the diet have taken this approach, but most people have stuck with two or three small meals per day.

The Shangri-La diet works by itself, but if you are already on another diet plan feel free to continue it. The Shangri-La diet may help you stick with it.

What to Expect

Most people who try the Shangri-La diet notice changes within a few days, others almost always within a week. Based on the many blog postings, e-mails, and phone calls I have received from happy dieters, the first changes include:

- *Less hunger.* "Tried this diet for 2 days and I am not as hungry as I usually am." After just a few days: "It makes you feel so stuffed. Unbelievable."

- *Feel full sooner.* At meals, you will stop eating after less food. "This is the first time I have ever left food on a plate," "I'm able to feel full after eating about half of what I normally eat," and "I was a three slices guy; now one slice of pizza is enough," are typical comments. To eat the amounts you used to eat will become unpleasant. "I went to a buffet with friends last week and ate more than I meant to. . . . I felt really bloated afterward," wrote one Shangri-La dieter.

- *Think about food less.* One of my students tried the diet not because she wanted to lose weight but because she wanted to think about food less often. She carefully measured how often she thought about food before and during the diet. She was skeptical, she said, but it worked.

- *Fewer cravings.* A woman told me that for many years she had uncontrollable night eating. "I would wake up and crave something to eat, fall asleep, wake up and crave something to eat and so on. I would snack as much as three times during my sleeping time," she said. "I never slept through the night, never." The first night after she began the Shangri-La diet, it stopped. "I have gotten the best sleep in I can't tell you how long," she said.

- *Better food choices.* The Shangri-La diet is like power steering: It helps you do what you want to do. One dieter put it like this: "[Before the diet] I would say I'm not going to eat something sweet—and I would give in and feel bad about myself. . . . Now I eat an apple and I'm done. . . . I'm in control and I'm making the right decisions rather than the food is in control of me." Another person said: "It's true that 400 or 500 calories of oil/sugar consists of empty calories, but it has replaced, easily, about 1,000 calories of junk—soda, cookies, candy, chips. . . . Before, I could not resist the junk."

See "In Shangri-La," pages 90–97, for more examples of these changes.

Soon after your hunger goes down, you will start to lose weight. Most people start losing weight within the first week. People often lose weight rather quickly at first (more than 2 pounds per week for a week or so), but then the weight loss slows down.

In one of my experiments, one subject, a young man, did not start losing weight until seven weeks had passed. When the diet portion of the experiment began, he was slowly gaining weight, so it took longer for him to start losing weight than if his weight had been steady. A friend of mine doing the diet took the "you can eat anything" rule to mean that he could now eat fattening foods, such as ice cream, that he had previously avoided. He started eating much more of these foods at the same time he started the diet. He did not gain weight—as he would have pre–Shangri-La—but he didn't lose weight either. The problem was that the amounts of sugar water and oil he was taking weren't large enough to overcome the increase in fattening foods.

Adjust the amount of sugar water and/or oil so that you lose no more than two pounds per week. If you are losing weight too quickly, cut back on the total number of calories you get from the sugar water and oil until your weight loss slows.

Now and then, your weight loss may stop for a week or so; this is mysterious but common. If your appetite *remains* low, it means that you will probably resume losing weight later. Simply continue with the same dose of sugar water and oil you have been using.

If your weight loss stops and your appetite *returns*, and you want to lose more weight, try either or both of these two things:

- Increase your dose of sugar water and/or oil by 100 calories a day (but do not exceed 400 calories per day total).

- Use the methods I describe in Chapter 6, "Extra Credit: Six More Ways to Lose Weight."

Almost everyone who does the diet has found that they need to adjust the dosage (sometimes up, sometimes down) to reach and stay at the weight they want.

Remember: *If you stop taking the sugar and/or oil, you will slowly regain the lost weight.* However, once you've reached your goal weight, you can skip days sometimes. If you find yourself regaining weight, just increase the dose on the days you do take it.

Possible Problems

Because the Shangri-La diet involves foods that are very common, it is almost always well tolerated. There is an important exception, however: people who have gallstones or who have had their gall-bladder removed usually are advised to avoid fatty foods. If you have gallbladder trouble or no longer have one, be cautious with the oil. Start with very small amounts (one teaspoon per day) that you gradually increase. Cut back or stop if digestive upset occurs. Or use sugar water instead.

Other minor problems sometimes occur:

- *Difficulty drinking oil.* It may help to take very small sips at first. There is no need to drink the oil all at once. It may also help to take a drink of water afterward.

- *Headache.* This is common. It is probably caused by suddenly consuming less sugar or caffeine than usual in your meals and snacks—for example, less chocolate, less soda, less junk food. The headaches usually go away after a few days or a week.

- *Too little flavor.* You may find yourself desiring flavor—not calories, just taste. "I still have a lot of mouth-boredom/antsiness and want to just put something in there," wrote one dieter. As I mentioned in Chapter 2, "The Case of the Missing Appetite," I dealt with this by drinking tea, chewing gum, and eating supermarket samples.

- *Stomach ache.* A few people have said that the fructose gave them a stomachache. If this happens, use sucrose instead.

- *Diarrhea.* Too much fructose at once can cause diarrhea. Be sure to drink it slowly.

- *More hunger than usual.* A few people have reported that the sugar water made them very hungry ("within thirty minutes, I was ravenously hungry"). If this happens, use the oil instead. This reaction may reflect a problem with how you metabolize sugar and is something to discuss with your doctor.

∽ Teacher and Student

TOM ROGERS, my brother-in-law, teaches journalism at San Jose State University. He learned about the weight-loss effects of ELOO at our Thanksgiving dinner in 2004. At the time, he weighed 178 pounds; he wanted to weigh in the mid-160s. (He is five foot ten.) He started with one tablespoon of ELOO per day. At Christmas, he heard me say something about two tablespoons per day, so he increased his intake to that amount. He drank all of it in the morning. He lost weight slowly. He found he no longer had to eat between meals. Or, if he really felt he must eat something, he'd just eat a few almonds and would feel fine. In the past, he'd gone to the kitchen and eaten a lot more than a few almonds. He also found he was eating smaller meals—perhaps 30 percent smaller. He got down to 170 in March and then increased the olive oil to three tablespoons per day in order to get to 166, which he reached in June 2005. He has stayed there for seven months. He goes on and off the olive oil; if he finds himself gaining weight, he starts taking it again. The best thing about the diet, he says, is that "you know you are not going to be overpowered by hunger so it is very easy to limit food intake. You are not fighting with hunger as you normally do on a diet."

Devon is a twenty-year-old student at a liberal arts college. She learned about the Shangri-La diet from *The New York Times*. She is five foot five; and when she began the diet, she weighed 238 pounds. She had gained weight every year and there seemed to be nothing she could do about it. For two months, she has been drinking one tablespoon of ELOO twice a day (two tablespoons per day), one in the morning and one in the afternoon, plus one tablespoon of sugar in one liter of water three times per day (three tablespoons per day).

Devon has lost thirteen pounds so far. Her eating has become much healthier. "Tonight, I went to the campus café," she told me, "and I saw a bag of baby carrots and thought, *Ooh, that sounds good,* and got them. That's new to me." In a funny way, the diet has given her permission to eat healthy food. If she feels like something sweet, she says, "I know this diet doesn't have any restrictions. So I'm telling myself to have a piece of fruit, and then if I still want the sweet thing I'll have it." At meals, she gets full a lot sooner. She still likes sweets but is no longer "addicted." She feels much more in control of what she eats. At first her friends thought the diet was crazy. "They are starting to think it's a lot less crazy," she said, "because they see how differently I'm eating."

Devon's view of herself has changed too. "I'm not so hard on myself when I do eat sweet stuff. Because I've eaten so healthily the rest of the day, when I eat something sweet I've earned it." She walks around campus more. She takes the stairs instead of the elevator. "I see how people who are fit walk up stairs without being out of breath. That's how I want to be."

5

COMMON QUESTIONS

I'VE BEEN asked about the diet by friends, students, Shangri-La bloggers, and others. Here are answers to the most common questions.

Technique

[Q] *Is extra-light-tasting olive oil the same as extra-light olive oil?*

[A] Yes. Extra-light olive oil (also known as extra-light-tasting olive oil) is barely colored. Extra-virgin olive oil is greenish, and because it has flavor, it will not work.

[Q] *What temperature should the sugar water be?*

[A] It doesn't matter. When I am cold, I find that hot sugar water is easy to drink. When I am warm (for instance, after exercise), cold sugar water is easy to drink. Room temperature is okay too. Hot water makes the sugar dissolve faster than cold water, and it has the added benefit of forcing you to drink it slowly, which helps avoid a blood sugar spike.

[Q] *How many sugar packets are in one tablespoon?*
[A] Sugar packets come in at least two sizes. For the smaller size, about four packets = one tablespoon; for the larger size, about three packets = one tablespoon. In my limited experience, cafés usually have the smaller size; supermarkets usually sell the larger size.

[Q] *Can I drink the oil or sugar water at bedtime?*
[A] Yes. Because you should not eat for an hour after you drink it, bedtime is a good time to take it.

[Q] *After I drink the oil or sugar water, I know I have to wait an hour before eating, but do I also need to wait an hour before having coffee/tea/ diet soda?*
[A] Yes, at least in the beginning. After it is clear that the diet is working, you can try relaxing this rule a bit (say, waiting only a half hour). If the diet stops working, you have relaxed the rule too much. The more closely you follow the rules, the better the diet is likely to work.

[Q] *I just brushed my teeth with mint toothpaste. Should I wait an hour before drinking the sugar water or oil?*

[A] Yes. The purpose of the one-hour rule is to prevent flavor-calorie associations from forming, and mint toothpaste has flavor. Again, once it is clear that the diet is working, you can try relaxing this rule a bit. If the diet stops working, you have relaxed the rule too much.

[Q] *When I drink the sugar water or olive oil, can I eat something else at the same time?*
[A] No. You must wait at least an hour before eating other food.

[Q] *Can I skip a day?*
[A] Yes. Skipping a day once every few weeks will have little effect.

[Q] *How often should I weigh myself?*
[A] It doesn't matter. The real signs that the diet is working will be that you feel less hungry than usual, that you snack less, that you eat less at meals, and that you think about food less often.

[Q] *Is exercise necessary?*
[A] Well, don't start exercising *less* than usual. Simply continue whatever exercise you already do. If you want to exercise more than usual, that's fine, and it will help you lose weight (and has other benefits as well), but it isn't necessary for success on this diet.

[Q] *Can I still do Weight Watchers?*

[A] Yes. For a class project, one of my students tried Weight Watchers. Her Weight Watchers plan assigned points to each food and allowed her to eat a certain number of points per week. After a few weeks, she found it hard to stay within the allotted points. She discovered that just two tablespoons of sugar in water per day made it much easier to stick with the plan. The friends with whom she had started Weight Watchers dropped out, but she continued, and by the end of class was still losing weight.

[Q] *Can I still do South Beach?*

[A] Yes. I originally planned to include a chapter about the good features of other popular diets, including South Beach. The top three good features of South Beach are:

- You eat new foods—foods with unfamiliar flavors not yet associated with calories. (As the new foods become familiar, however, the diet becomes less effective.)

- You eat fewer ditto foods—foods that taste exactly the same each time—because you cook more, and much of the ditto food you usually eat is forbidden (e.g., junk food).

- You stop eating food with a high glycemic index, such as white bread and potatoes.

These three changes lower your set point. The next chapter, "Extra Credit: Six More Ways to Lose Weight," discusses each of them at length.

[Q] *Are you telling me that I have to drink sugar water or olive oil every day for the rest of my life?*

[A] No. After you reach your target weight, you may be able to reduce how much sugar water and/or oil you consume. One way to reduce the dose is to skip days, as Sarah did (see Figure 4 on page 38). However, you must continue to take the sugar water or oil at least some of the time, as Tom Rogers does ("Teacher and Student" interlude, pages 78–80)—or else you will slowly regain the lost weight.

Substitutions

[Q] *Can I use a noncaloric or low-calorie sweetener (such as aspartame or stevia) instead of sugar?*

[A] No. The sugar water and oil cause you to lose weight because they provide calories without raising your set point. Water sweetened with a no-calorie sweetener doesn't do that. Water sweetened with a low-calorie sweetener barely does, and as a result is barely effective.

[Q] *Can I use honey instead of sugar?*

[A] Some Shangri-La dieters have tried honey in place of sugar, with mixed results. It works for some people but not for others. If the flavor of the honey is new to you, it should work until the flavor becomes associated with calories. If the flavor is mild, that might take a while. Even then, the final flavor-calorie association may be weak because fructose, the main sugar in honey, is digested slowly. If you want to try honey, it's a good idea to begin with regular sugar. After you've gotten the diet working with regular sugar water, switch to honey water and see if it continues to work. To reduce flavor, you should dilute the honey quite a bit—use at least two cups of water per tablespoon of honey. If you start thinking the honey water tastes good, that's a bad sign, because it means your body has learned to associate the honey flavor with calories. If the honey flavor becomes associated with calories, it will raise your set point.

[Q] *What about olive oil–filled gel caps?*
[A] Yes, you can use them. But it isn't easy. A large gel cap will contain 1,000 mg of olive oil, which has only 9 calories. To get 300 calories per day, you must swallow thirty-three gel caps per day.

[Q] *Can I drink flax oil instead of canola/ safflower/extra-light olive oil?*
[A] Maybe. I tried two different brands of flax oil. Both worked, as far as I could tell. But flax oil seems to me more flavorful than ELOO, canola oil, or safflower oil. Perhaps its flavor will eventually become associated with calories. Another disadvantage of flax oil is that it is much more expensive than the other oils, about forty cents for 100 calories.

Why It Works

[Q] *Why doesn't the body learn to associate the sweetness of sugar with calories?*

[A] I don't know. Maybe because sweetness plays a different dietary role than other flavors. Sweetness has the curious feature that sweet foods taste *worse* when we are hungry than when we are not hungry. All plants contain sugar; maybe we like sweetness so that we will eat more plants. Or maybe we don't associate sweetness with calories because sweetness is so common that we come to ignore it, just as we stop noticing a persistent noise.

[Q] *Does the Shangri-La diet work by decreasing appetite or increasing metabolism?*

[A] Short answer: Decreasing appetite. Your metabolism slows down as you lose weight. Long answer: Neither. It works by lowering your set point. It will usually take a month or more before your decreasing weight catches up with your decreasing set point. When that happens, your appetite will return. But it's still working because your set point is still much lower than when you started.

Health Concerns

[Q] *Does sugar water cause cavities?*

[A] I asked Norman Temple, a professor of nutrition at Athabasca University, in Athabasca, Canada, and co-editor of *Beverages in Nutrition and Health*

(2002). He said that although sugar-containing foods cause cavities, the problem is the sticky foods, not sugar water. "With sugary water, it doesn't hang around in the mouth long enough, it doesn't stick to the teeth like candy. Your saliva dilutes it quickly. It can very easily get diluted and washed away by the saliva. So there is very little time for the sugar to be metabolized by the bacteria in the mouth, produce acid, and then start eating away at the enamel." The more diluted your sugar water (the more water per tablespoon of sugar), the less sugar is available to the bacteria.

[Q] *I have a family history of diabetes. Is this diet safe for me?*
[A] Safety questions should be answered by your doctor, who will take your medical history into consideration. If you're diabetic, you should choose to drink the oil, which will not affect your blood sugar levels.

If you are concerned about developing diabetes, keep in mind that the risk of diabetes increases sharply with weight. In one study, persons with a body mass index (BMI) of more than 35 were eighty times more likely to get diabetes than a person with a BMI of 22 or less. Another study found that women with a BMI between 23 and 24 (which is not even considered overweight) were four times more likely to get diabetes than women with a BMI of less than 21. An experiment in Finland with persons on the edge of getting diabetes found that lifestyle changes that caused them to lose ten pounds reduced their chances of becoming diabetic during the next four years by 60 percent. (Many websites, such as nhlbisupport.com/bmi, will calculate your BMI for you.)

General

[Q] *What about emotional eating?*
[A] This is a hard question to answer. What I've seen is that this diet helps people control their cravings, eat less, and make food choices that they themselves consider to be better. I think the jury is still out on whether the diet reduces eating that's due to frustration or stress.

[Q] *Is this another fad diet?*
[A] Well, the Shangri-La diet is based on scientific research (see the Appendix, "The Science Behind the Theory Behind the Diet," pages 141–157) much more than most previous diets. Science has often provided better solutions than other problem-solving methods.

∼ In Shangri-La

But here, at Shangri-La, all was in deep calm.
—*Lost Horizon*

As THE introduction says, I decided to call this book *The Shangri-La Diet* because many people said the diet greatly reduced their struggles with food. Here are some examples from conversations, e-mails, and blog postings:

"Before this, I felt powerless over food. Diets never worked. It was just an addiction: I can't stop eating sweets, can't stop eating crappy food. Now I eat when I'm hungry."

"It's great to feel like I'm in control of things. Before my appetite was driving me; after eating I'd feel angry and guilty."

"I never eat the sweets at lunch anymore. Rarely at dinner. Now I'll look at something and think: If that's all they have and it's not that good, what's the point?"

"I just don't have that craving where I'm drawn to the refrigerator or wherever I have food and just start eating. . . . I'm not finding that happening [now that I'm drinking] the sugar water. It helps me resist temptation."

"[My] weight gain over the years had little to do with being hungry, but more [with] the reckless need to eat fattening foods such as bread and butter, dishes with cream sauces, cheese, ice cream, pastries and the like; it was more like an addiction to fat and carbohydrates. Following your recommendations helps control those urges, or perceived needs for "bad" things. . . . On Saturday I treated myself to light ice cream, and was perfectly content with 2 scoops (1 cup) for 240 calories."

"I saw the segment on GMA [Good Morning America] this morning. . . . I had gone to the gym at around six and had dinner around 7:30. I usually eat something else before I go to bed (popcorn, cheese) and I could feel the post dinner evening cravings setting in. I bit the bullet and swallowed a tablespoon of [canola] oil. Greasy but tasteless. Quite honestly, my cravings and desire to eat completely evaporated. 100%! And people, this never, ever happens to me."

"The most enormous difference I can see [since starting the diet a week ago] is that junk food—which used to sing its high-calorie, over-processed siren song to me loud and long, day in and day out—now holds only minimal appeal."

"I like cookies, and they are available at work. That's my problem. In these first two days, when I got the urge for some cookies, I drank the water.

That meant I drank a couple of tablespoons of fructose per day instead of eating a dozen cookies. . . . The net effect has been I've eaten much less sugar."

"I used to snack all day. In particular, chocolate. There's a steady supply around the office. But since I started this I've stopped eating the chocolate. . . . It simply doesn't occur to me to impulsively walk over and grab some, as I used to."

"My interest in chocolate has dropped dramatically—not completely, but dramatically. I generally keep a bag of little chocolate things around, like chocolate kisses. I'd go through a 2 lb. bag of Hershey's Nuggets in a couple of weeks. I'm going through them much less than half as fast."

"The sugar water seems to be doing away with most of my cravings thus far (it's only been two days)."

"Since I have been doing this, my between-meal cravings have all disappeared, and for the first time in my life I can look at something like popcorn, chocolate, potato chips, french fries, etc., and say 'I'm not hungry' and pass it up."

"It's just amazing how much my desire to snack has gone down. Don't have a whole lot of interest in it."

"I didn't realize to what extent my nighttime cravings were taking over. Now I come home and I just don't feel the need to snack."

"The best part of it is the snacking is cut out. Used to be a snacking frenzy at home after work while I'm cooking."

"I essentially cut all starches out of my diet permanently (I thought) because I just couldn't control myself around bread, cookies, bagels, etc. . . . Now, suddenly, I can eat a small amount of those things and not fall down the rabbit hole. Hallelujah."

"My weakness before the program was junky carbs—pretzels, breads, and the like. I noticed in the first week or two that my desire for carbs was significantly diminished."

"A few weeks ago I would have made a beeline [to the new Starbucks]. Now I'm just vaguely interested in perhaps going there to sit. . . . It is such a relief! I can still eat delicious things, but I'm definitely no longer entranced."

"This Thursday will make 1 full week since I've tried it. . . . I still eat 'regular food' but I have no cravings, and I end up eating a whole lot less as a result. . . . When I get home, I'm not famished and don't overeat."

"I started [six days ago]. . . . I was amazed at how quickly my appetite was under control. I say under control because I still ate but did not have constant cravings."

"I avoid desserts and overeating far more than before the fructose. It's the fructose taking away that hunger edge that allows me to avoid them. 8 years of trying to cut them out didn't work, but the fructose did."

"I have used the oil for a week now. It has changed my appetite. I was one of those that ate something salty and then had a need for something sweet and so on. It was like a never ending circle of cravings. I no longer have those needs to snack and cover the taste of the previous snack."

"Last week a neighbor dropped off a piece of chocolate cake and it actually went stale. I forgot it was there. Unheard of. . . . There is no willpower involved here. I still don't have any willpower. I'm just not hungry for those things."

THE SHANGRI-LA diet has reduced eating at night:

"[Before this diet, I] would sometimes wake up at midnight and eat 500–1,000 calories (sometimes more). . . . I have not eaten anything after dinner since I started six weeks ago, and not felt like I wanted or needed to."

"*I became a night eater. I developed a habit—even when I fell asleep, I would wake up and crave something to eat, fall asleep, wake up and crave something to eat and so on. I would snack as much as 3 times during my sleeping time. . . . For the past week between 9:00–10:00 p.m., I take a teaspoon of EVOO.* [Author's note: I suggest ELOO rather than EVOO; EVOO may eventually stop working.] *Believe it or not, my hunger is gone during the night and I have gotten the best sleep in I can't tell you how long.*"

"*I like to measure time by how long it takes to finish a box of Yodels. But I didn't even think about eating them. Normally I would eat them at night but I didn't. I forgot about them.*"

"*The diet works, it's easy, I eat whatever I feel like, but I snack much much less, no late night noshing, and I don't miss it.*"

"*I do fine during the day—it's in the evening that I have the snacking problem. I will say the hot sugar water does seem to remove my cravings.*"

"*No more late-night snacking, when I used to pop a bunch of cookies or crackers or cheese things. No chip cravings. It's the junk I've cut out.*"

THE SHANGRI-LA diet has allowed people to think about food less:

"The constant thoughts I have about eating have subsided. One of the problems I have always had is that my brain is constantly thinking about food . . . what I'm eating, when I will eat, where I will eat and what I'm eating at the next meal, etc."

"I'm eating to live rather than the other way around."

"I'm so grateful for not thinking about food all the time."

"I have been able to stop thinking about food during times when I need to be working, cleaning, or playing."

THE DIET has made it easier to make good food choices:

"When I do decide to eat, I choose things that are good for me. No more junk food."

"I am able to make good decisions about how much I need to eat to keep my body going."

"[Before this diet] I would say I'm not going to eat something sweet—but then I would give in and feel bad about myself or I wouldn't and would be tortured by it. Now I eat an apple and I'm done. . . . I'm

in control and I'm making the right decisions rather than the food is in control of me."

SOME SHANGRI-LA dieters say it has given them more appreciation of food:

"I was seeing food as a negative thing because I kept gaining weight. Now I'm seeing it as the positive thing it is."

"When I eat sweets I enjoy it so much more—I savor it, because I'm not eating it all the time. I appreciate the richness of it."

6

EXTRA CREDIT: SIX MORE WAYS TO LOSE WEIGHT

SUGAR WATER and/or flavorless oil between meals should take you many pounds below your starting weight, painlessly. It may well allow you to lose all the weight you want to lose, as happened to me, my brother-in-law, and others.

But you may want to lose even more weight. Or lose weight more quickly. Or reduce the amount of sugar water or oil you take. (As one blogger wrote, "Not sure I look forward to a lifetime of sugar water or oil between meals.") Fortunately, the theory that led me to discover the effects of sugar water and oil (see Chapter 3, "A New Theory of Weight Loss") suggests many other ways to lose weight, six of which I describe in this chapter. Each one is a different way to lower your set point. You might think of them as extra credit—not required but helpful.

All six methods are based on the same basic principle: Foods with strong flavor-calorie associations are more fattening than foods with weak flavor-calorie associations; this is because they raise your set point more. And, for the same reason, foods with weak flavor-calorie associations are more fattening than foods with no flavor-calorie association.

Method 1. Try new foods.

Foods with new flavors have no flavor-calorie association. Trying new foods can be as simple as buying new foods. In Paris, I lost weight because I drank new soft drinks. I like jams and jellies, but I avoid buying the same flavor twice. Rather than buy the same old frozen entrée, try a new one. Try a new flavor of soup. At a restaurant, order something new.

Restaurants with varying menus and daily specials make this easy. In *French Women Don't Get Fat*, Mireille Guiliano writes that "my business requires me to eat in restaurants about three hundred times a year." If these three hundred meals are at many different fancy restaurants whose menus change frequently, it is quite possible she rarely eats the same thing twice. Could this be why she has stayed slim? Dorie Greenspan, author of *Paris Sweets*, a cookbook about Paris pastries, told an interviewer that she's "always thought the [real] French Paradox is the way thin French women eat dessert three times a day [at cafés] and they're still thin." If they eat many different desserts at many different cafés—easy to do in Paris—this is no paradox.

The notion that novelty matters is new to the world of diets. At calorielab.com, an independent website about nutrition and weight loss, a blogger wrote, "I think we can say with a certain amount of confidence that things like the Starbucks 730-calorie Venti Caramel Chocolate Frappuccino with whipped cream fall outside the Shangri-La Diet." Well, no, not the *first* time you have it. Having it *once* is fine. This is not idle speculation. Recently I went to a special dinner celebrating the day on which James Joyce's novel *Ulysses* takes place (Bloomsday, June 16th). Most of the dishes at the dinner were Irish, such as corned beef and cabbage. Dessert, though, was Italian: tiramisu, usually made with eggs, sugar, mascarpone, espresso, cocoa, and brandy or marsala. The Bloomsday version, however, used Baileys Irish Cream as the liquor. The portions were big; my piece probably had several hundred calories. But it tasted unfamiliar. I had had tiramisu many times. I had had Baileys Irish Cream many times. In spite of this, their combination was unfamiliar, which meant it qualified as new food. The next day I had remarkably little appetite and ate very little—due to the unusual tiramisu, I'm sure. The Baileys tiramisu was the opposite of fattening: It lowered my set point. This made me less hungry than usual the next day, so I ate less than usual.

Support for the idea that new-flavored foods

cause weight loss can be found in *The Flavor Point Diet* by Dr. David Katz. The diet consists of eating only one flavor per meal without any calorie restriction. In practice, Flavor Point dieters eat almost nothing but new foods with unusual flavors. And it works, at least for a while: In twelve weeks, dieters lost an average of 17 pounds. The book has no data about what happens after that—when the new foods become familiar.

Method 2. Cook more.

The opposite of new food is familiar food; and the foods that can become most familiar are those that taste exactly the same each time—what I call ditto foods. These mass-produced foods come mostly from factories and chain restaurants. Because their flavors are so constant, when they are eaten repeatedly they can produce very strong flavor-calorie associations—much stronger than similar foods that vary in flavor, such as your homemade lasagna or meat loaf, which vary a bit each time you make them. (To increase the power of this method, I intentionally vary the flavors of my cooking.)

Ditto foods are the profit centers of the food industry. They include convenience food (such as frozen entrées, breakfast cereals, canned and frozen juices), ready-to-eat food, canned soup, junk food (such as soda, potato chips, and candy), fast food, and chain restaurant food. Almost any food sold in a package or made in a factory qualifies. It isn't just "bad" food; "good" food can be ditto food as well. "I've been having granola and soy milk for breakfast every day for months," wrote a woman who was trying my diet. "At first it made me extremely full until lunchtime. Now I'm hungry within a couple of hours." No doubt the granola was manufactured rather than homemade and tasted the same each time. And the soy milk tasted exactly the same each time. When she first started to eat the granola/soy milk combination, it was unfamiliar to her, and it acted like sugar water and flavorless oil: it lowered her set point. But with time, the flavors became associated with calories and became fattening. Chapter 7, "Changing the Rest of the World," explains why I believe the cause of today's obesity epidemic is an increase in the consumption of ditto foods—or, to put it another way, a decrease in home cooking.

Home cooks are neither machines nor fast-food restaurant employees following precise instructions with ingredients that are always the same. This is why a home-cooked dish usually varies from one rendition to the next far more than factory food or fast food. "The most successful dieters, we've found," observes Dr. Arthur Agatston in *The South Beach Diet,* "are the ones who try every recipe imaginable and take advantage of all the foods and ingredients permitted. . . . One patient invented a new soup made with every green vegetable he could find." The flavor of this soup surely varied a lot from one batch to the next. (And by trying new recipes, Dr. Agatston's most successful dieters were also following Method 1, "Try new food.") Leftovers, unfortunately, are ditto food; so when you cook, make only enough for one meal.

Only foods that always taste the same become addictive. For example, a *New Yorker* article in 1995 by Susan Sheehan described an Iowa family that was living near poverty and seemingly headed toward bankruptcy. To save the price of a stamp, they paid bills in person. Yet the husband and wife both drank a lot of Pepsi every day, calling themselves "Pepsiholics." Almost every week, they ate dinner at McDonald's. "Going out to dinner is as necessary to me as paying water bills," said the husband. Other ditto foods produce similar behavior. As a high-school student, Jill Ciment wrote in her lovely memoir, *Half a Life*, she deeply wanted to save money to go to New York. She took on extra jobs, but couldn't manage to save anything. "I wasn't wanton with my money. . . . I just felt the dire need to reward myself for all my dogged hard work, to splurge on the extra candy bar, the jumbo Coke." When In-N-Out Burger, a California chain, opened a new store in 1996, one of the first customers was a college student majoring in health education. "I was such a fan, I [had been] driving to Atascadero whenever I could convince somebody it was worth a three-hour drive," he told a reporter. "Now we have one here, and I'm in heaven."

Pepsi, McDonald's, candy bars, Coke, In-N-Out burgers—all ditto foods. Dr. William Jacobs, a professor of psychiatry at the University of Florida's

College of Medicine, told me that the food addicts he has seen have usually been addicted to commercial soft drinks, ice cream, and certain fast foods, such as pizza and hamburgers—again, all ditto food. He never saw anyone addicted to homemade hamburgers or homemade pizza. He also encountered persons addicted to iced tea (with lots of sugar). The iced tea was both commercial and homemade; iced tea is so simple to make that even prepared at home it can taste exactly the same each time (especially if you use a mix). Addictive foods are addictive because they produce great pleasure. They do so because of a very strong flavor-calorie association. To build up a very strong flavor-calorie association, the flavor needs to be exactly the same each time you eat the food.

Method 3. Add random flavors.

An unusual way to vary the flavor of your food is to *add several randomly chosen flavors.* One way to do this is to have many different flavor shakers, each with a different spice—basil, cumin, cinnamon, coriander, dill, garlic powder, ginger, mustard, paprika, pepper, nutmeg, oregano, and thyme—and season your food with a few of them, randomly selected. Because the combination will be different every time, it will never become familiar. Dr. Alan Hirsch, a Chicago neurologist, did a study that suggests this will work. He gave subjects flavorings to sprinkle on all of their food: two flavors each month for six months. Cheddar cheese (for savory foods) and cocoa (for sweet foods) were the first two, onion (savory) and spearmint (sweet) the next two, horseradish (savory) and banana (sweet) after that, and so on. Because the foods on which these flavorings were sprinkled already had flavor, this must have produced many novel flavor combinations. The novelty continued because the flavors changed every month. During the six-month experiment, the subjects lost an average of thirty-four pounds. Control subjects followed a traditional diet program and gained a small amount of weight.

You can take the first steps in this direction by simply adding a variety of seasonings to whatever ditto foods you eat. Instead of tasting exactly the same each time, these foods will now taste different each time, and as a result will be less fattening. In Chapter 7, on prevention, I discuss this approach at greater length. This method surprises many people, so let me be clear: I *am* saying that if you add cinnamon to your pizza it will make it less fattening, at least the first time you do it.

Method 4. Eat one food at a time.

My theory predicts that some foods are fattening because of what they combine; their ingredients eaten separately would not be fattening. I have eaten my share of pastrami sandwiches, for example. They taste very good to me because of the pastrami flavor. This is a sign that the pastrami flavor has become strongly associated with calories. Yet the average pastrami sandwich doesn't have many calories of pastrami. When I eat a pastrami sandwich, the pastrami and mustard produce a strong flavor signal; the bread, which has quickly digested calories, produces a large and quick calorie signal. The combination of the two produces a strong flavor-calorie association (see Chapter 3, "A New Theory of Weight Loss," for explanation). Pastrami eaten alone would not do this: It doesn't produce a strong fast calorie signal. The bread eaten alone would not do this: It doesn't have a strong flavor. Because pastrami alone and bread alone would produce weaker flavor-calorie associations, eating them separately (pastrami at 1 p.m., bread at 2 p.m.) would be less fattening—that is, would raise my set point less—than eating them together. (I don't actually do this; it is just a simple example to make the point.) With a pastrami sandwich, the meat and the bread happen to be two parts of the same dish. The general idea is that two dishes on one plate—roast beef and mashed potatoes, for instance—can act in the same way. By eating dishes at separate times, there is less of what I call *cross-conditioning,* and the flavor-calorie associations that develop are weaker.

This method of weight loss has been discovered by people not armed with my theory. It has an odd name: *food combining. Food separating* would be more descriptive, because it has rules such as "Do not eat fats with proteins" and "Do not consume starch and sugars together." The idea may have come to public attention in the bestselling book *Fit for Life* (1985) by Harvey and Marilyn Diamond.

Suzanne Somers's popular diet books take this approach as well. I'm sure it works; it's just too hard to sustain. An Italian friend of mine went to a diet expert in Milan and was given a weight-loss plan that allowed only one type of food per meal. Monday lunch: vegetables. Monday dinner: protein. Tuesday lunch: fruit. And so on. It was very effective. Over five months, my friend lost about seventy pounds. Then he slowly gained it back, because the diet was too difficult. Four years later, he started the diet again and re-lost about seventy pounds. Then he re-fell off the wagon and slowly regained the lost weight. Quitting smoking is *much* easier than dieting, he says.

Less extreme versions of this approach are helpful, I believe. The French eat different dishes at different times during a meal. The vegetable dish is eaten separately from the meat dish, for example; the two courses might be separated by twenty minutes. This way of eating has the pleasant side effect of making meals easier to prepare, since there is no need to have several dishes ready at the same time.

Method 5. Eat foods that are digested slowly.

In Chapter 3, I discussed why food that is digested more slowly produces weaker flavor-calorie associations. In practice, until we can conveniently measure the calorie signals produced by fats and proteins, eating foods that are digested slowly means eating more foods with a low glycemic index

The Glycemic Index

A food's glycemic index (GI) tells you how quickly its carbohydrates are digested. High GI = Fast digestion. Low GI = Slow digestion. For foods that are mostly carbohydrate, the GI is a good measure of the speed of digestion. The GI values of many foods can be found at www.mendosa.com /gilists.htm. A searchable database is at www.glycemic index.com.

HIGH GI FOODS	LOW GI FOODS
Most bread	Dried apricots
Dates	Grapefruit
Rice Krispies	Cherries
Instant mashed potatoes	Black beans
Baked potato	Lentils

and fewer foods with a high glycemic index (see box, above). There are several good books about how to do this, such as *The New Glucose Revolution* (2003), by Jennie Brand-Miller and colleagues. As I mentioned earlier, when I did this I lost six pounds. This was not earth-shattering, but it was so easy to continue to eat this way that I never regained the lost weight.

Low-carb and good-carb diets work moderately well. I believe this is because they replace carbohydrates that are digested quickly (high glycemic index foods), such as bread, potatoes, and sweets, with foods that are digested more slowly, such as fats, proteins, and low glycemic index carbohydrates such as green vegetables. The slowly digested foods have weaker flavor-calorie associations than the quickly digested foods and thus raise your set point less.

Method 6. Eat foods with less flavor.

Weak flavors, like slowly digested foods, never become strongly associated with calories (see Chapter 3, page 46, for more on this). This makes foods with weak flavors—I'll call them *delicately flavored* foods—less fattening than other foods. It isn't easy to eat enough of these foods to lose significant amounts of weight. I tried to eat plain white fish—no seasonings at all—and gave up after one meal. Sushi was easier; I lost weight on my sushi diet. But it was hard to eat sushi day after day, not to mention expensive and unwise due to mercury in tuna. I believe that many meal-replacement drinks such as Slim-Fast are effective because they have weak

A FEW DELICATELY FLAVORED FOODS

Cottage cheese

Plain tofu

White rice

Cod and other white fish

Nigiri sushi (raw fish on white rice) without wasabi

flavors. They replace foods with stronger flavors. Much cheaper delicately flavored foods are widely available (see box, "A Few Delicately Flavored Foods," page 109).

While it is hard to eat food with little flavor, it is quite possible to eat food with *less* flavor. "I just leave off some salt, sweetener or sauce that I would usually use," one Shangri-La dieter wrote. "Next thing you know, I can't finish the plate of food. I can't live on bland, but once in a while it's a big help."

Behind the sugar water and oil of Shangri-La Basic is the idea that the most potent weight-loss foods are those with *no* flavor. Timothy Beneke, an Oakland, California, writer, used this idea in a new way. In 1999, he weighed 280 pounds. His doctor told him he was nearly diabetic. Strongly motivated by this news, he used my early weight-loss methods (eat less-processed foods, low glycemic index foods, and weakly flavored foods) to go from 280 to 250 pounds. When I told him that I had lost weight drinking fructose water, he started drinking it too. By drinking six tablespoons of fructose per day, he lost about fifty pounds in nine months. At two hundred pounds, however, he started regaining weight. I warned him that overshoot—more weight loss than can ultimately be sustained, as mentioned in Chapter 4, "How to Do the Shangri-La Diet"—was possible on the Shangri-La diet, but he interpreted the regain to mean that the sugar water had stopped working. He stopped drinking it, and his weight went back up to 250 pounds.

After I told Tim about the good results I had with extra-light olive oil, he tried it. By drinking three tablespoons of ELOO a day, he lost weight steadily, reaching 210 pounds. At that point, his appetite returned and he had trouble staying at that weight. But he did not want to increase his daily amount of ELOO or resume the sugar water.

To provide a nutritious source of more flavorless calories, Tim inventively combined "liquefied fruits and vegetables, mixed with a powder made of brown rice, almond meal, flaxseed meal, dry nonfat milk, garbanzo powder, potato flour, and soy protein powder" (this description is from his web posting). He cooked the mixture until it was thick enough to make small clumps, then used a little spoon to form little pellets, which he swallowed with water as if they were pills. He simply ate some of this whenever he felt hungry, enough to make the hunger go away. He also ate normally (ordinary restaurant food, for instance) and continued to drink ELOO.

The mush worked, in the sense that Tim did not regain the weight he had already lost. "Doing 25% of my calories with mush and olive oil only kept me at 210 for 10 months," he wrote. But he didn't lose any more weight. Then, after ten months, he increased the mush to about 75 percent of his calories and found that he started losing weight again. Over five months, he went from 210 to 180 pounds, which he was pleased with. As of December 2005, he has stayed at 180 for seven months, while getting about 40 percent of his calories from his mush clumps.

Tim Beneke used my theory in a new way to sustainably lose *more* weight after first using it to lose eighty pounds. This is excellent support for the theory. Because the methods of this chapter are based on the theory, the more we can believe the theory, the more we can believe that the methods will work.

Beneke's method is extreme, but it is has produced great results. It is certainly far better—cheaper, safer, more widely available, and probably more sustainable—than another extreme solution, gastric bypass surgery.

If I Had Two Hundred Pounds to Lose . . .

If I had two hundred pounds to lose, the first thing I'd try, in addition to the sugar water and oil, would be randomly flavoring all my foods, especially the ditto foods. I'd also cook as much as possible, replacing ditto food with homemade food and varying the spices. But the other methods have value too. I eat foods separately when possible; I have avoided high glycemic index foods for many years; I enjoy sushi now and then; and when a unique dessert comes my way, I eat it eagerly.

The Blogosphere Tries It

AFTER A *Freakonomics* column about the Shangri-La diet appeared in *The New York Times Magazine* (September 11, 2005), Stephen Dubner and Steven Levitt, the authors of the column, kindly invited me to guest-blog at www.freakonomics.com. Something unexpected happened: People started posting their experience with the diet. The very first report was negative:

> "I tried a tablespoon of extra-virgin olive oil yesterday and of canola oil today. . . . Neither one did anything for my hunger; I ate just as much as usual at my subsequent meals."

THEY SOON became overwhelmingly positive:

> "I don't need to lose weight but I must say this sugar water stuff works like magic for me."

> "Whoa. Close to zero appetite. . . . Ridiculously easy. And cheap. And effective. What hath God wrought?"

> "I've lost 6 lbs. in 5 days, despite eating better than I have in years. . . . For me, the debate is over. I've never been able to lose weight so effectively—not even

on a raw foods diet or when athletically swimming four hours a week."

"When I started this, I weighed 226. I now weigh 220.5. Not bad for 9 days. . . . My diet is as varied and as nutritious as ever, perhaps more so."

"I've lost about 3 pounds in ten days. Not earth shattering, but slow and steady is good I think."

"Your conclusions on fructose sugar are right on the money. I've got 20 lbs. of weight loss so far to prove it."

THERE WERE a few failures too:

"I tried fructose water for 3–4 days and GAINED THREE POUNDS!!! 45–60 minutes after drinking the sugar water I WAS RAVENOUS!!!"

"I've tried the regime for about two weeks now with no results. I've been drinking 250 calories of fructose dissolved in a liter of water. . . . I haven't gained weight, but I haven't lost any either."

BILL Q. wrote at freakonomics.com: "I've been on the diet for three days. I've lost seven pounds. I've not had a moment of hunger, nor have I experienced any odd cravings." He added that he would post later results at his blog "assuming the program is a success." No later results appeared, suggesting that the program failed.

After my freakonomics.com stint, Ann Hendricks set up Annie's Shangri-La Diet Blog (ann hendricksshangrila.blogspot.com) so that people trying the diet could share their experiences. As of January 2006, there are about two hundred posts. They tell the stories of nine people:

DE BENCI, starting at 185 pounds, lost eight pounds over eight weeks, making only changes "that I feel I can stick with in the long term." He successfully used honey water instead of sugar water.

EMILY started at 276 pounds. Over seven weeks, she lost fourteen pounds. "It is very interesting to feel like I might have some measure of control over my weight. Previously, I have tried the standard diet and exercise method and have felt hungry, deprived, and frustrated."

JULIE had little luck. She lost a few pounds at first but then stopped losing. Eventually, "I stopped drinking my sugar water because I didn't think it was working for me. I gained back the weight I lost."

LEFTBLANC started at 226 pounds. Over eleven weeks, he lost twenty-five pounds. (See page 121 for more about his experience.)

MASA'IL (Hendricks herself). Starting at 192 pounds, she was down to 176 pounds—eighteen pounds lost in eleven weeks. The diet, in her experience, is "definitely irreplaceable so far: Nothing [else] has helped me as much."

MICHELLE started at 170 pounds. Over five weeks, she lost fourteen pounds. "I'm definitely making better choices when I do eat," she wrote. "Food is still very appealing to me, but I'm drawn to good food and proper portions. It's not effortless or even particularly easy, but it does seem possible." She began to feel skeptical, yet still hopeful, after she skipped her Shangri-La routine for a few days and her hunger returned. However, getting back on the diet did not immediately curb her appetite.

MOLLY. After two weeks, she wrote: "Jeez, this diet makes me so hopeful it's almost scary. I've fought my weight my whole life, and the idea that I might actually be able to reach my ideal weight and stay there is . . . the word *miraculous* keeps coming to mind. No dangerous drugs? No diet restrictions like no carbs, or no fats? No grinding hunger? And I can eat and enjoy pleasurable foods? It boggles the mind." After three weeks, she had lost six pounds, and wrote: "So much of what I previously thought about weight loss, diet and nutrition seems useless in light of my experience on this diet." The most recent summary I have of her experience is: "I lost 12 pounds [in eight weeks, starting at 155], then went on vacation for 2 weeks and (stupidly) gained back 6, of which I have now re-lost 3 (in 4 days)." The diet "is a very useful tool for controlling eating while trying to lose weight," she wrote. "And I'm very grateful for that."

SARAH's first post said that she had been "doing the diet for almost 2 weeks. It is working like a dream. . . . I feel great, I've got energy to work out for more than an hour, and I am really, really excited that this is working so easily. I have lost about 4 lbs. and that is big since I am trying to lose the last 15 of a 100-lb. weight loss and before now, it just would not budge." She lost weight steadily. Three weeks later, in her last post, she wrote, "I have nothing to report except consistent, slightly boring weight loss with not a lot of effort—which of course is huge and un-precedented for me."

SFC started at 184 and over three months steadily lost eighteen pounds. "This has been nearly effort-less," he wrote. "My food cravings are down, my appetite is down, and I very, very seldom eat more than 2,000 calories a day, which before I started was more like my minimum calorie consumption." After he e-mailed me, I spoke to him by phone. He said he lost the weight without any exercise—a de-liberate choice. During the first eight weeks, he had drunk up to 500 calories per day of fructose water; then he switched to mostly extra-light olive oil. The oil worked as well as the fructose water.

THE RESULTS were so consistently positive that Hendricks eventually asked people to post other outcomes:

"Getting the real range of experiences posted would definitely be the best way to really explore this thing. . . . Any failures or 'less-than-spectacular successes'?"

AFTER THIS, two people posted:

ROBERT F. wrote that he had "tried the diet over the past two months with only minimal success." (I believe his dose of sugar water was not large enough to overcome his "resumption of eating carbs.")

AGNOSTIC wrote, "I lost 5 pounds in 3 weeks [but] I haven't lost any [more] weight for a month now."

SOON AFTER the *Freakonomics* column, calorielab. com, an independent website about nutrition and weight, posted a long article about the diet. Bottom line: "If you had to cook up the ultimate stereotype of a wacky fad diet for use in a comedic novel or film, the Shangri-La Diet would fill the bill." However, "we're not necessarily saying it won't work." The article discussed the ideas behind it, adding "we suspect he cooked it [the theory behind the diet] up as an afterthought to justify his development of a weight-loss program while being employed as a psychology professor." (Actually, the theory came first.) Then the success stories, posted as comments to the CalorieLab report, began:

> "*I am two weeks into the oil diet. . . . I have lost three pounds. Was 168. lbs, 5´11˝. . . . Appetite much suppressed. Not much determination required to take small helpings. Eating is oddly optional after a very small meal.*"

CALORIELAB noted that people eat for reasons other than hunger, thus "a system like Roberts's that supposedly suppresses actual gimme-energy hunger is not going to work long term, once the initial excitement of trying a new diet wears off." The successful dieter replied:

> "*Separating, through this diet, gimme-energy hunger from the other motivations to eat has been instructive. The other motivations are much clearer. . . . They are easier to control because the gimme-energy hunger is suppressed.*"

THE SUCCESS stories continued:

> "*I am 54, 5´8˝ post-menopausal at 146 lbs. I have been on this program for 10 days and have lost 4 pounds. . . . I am delighted with the current cut in appetite.*"

> "*I have been using the 'Shangri-la' diet now for almost a month, and it works beautifully. It has re-*

moved my cravings and registers a full stomach whenever I eat."

CALORIELAB replied: "Remember: The whole diet may be nonsense and not work." But then:

> "Have been doing this for 3 weeks. . . . Have lost 11 pounds and it's been easy."

> "I just have to say it works. I tried it for 2 weeks. . . . I have lost my extra fat around the waist I had after having 3 kids."

A *Good Morning America* segment about the diet on November 14 produced a burst of questions, which CalorieLab patiently answered, adding "we think this is just a crazy fad diet." The mini–success stories continued:

> "I've been following your Shangri La guidelines now for 3 days. . . . It does appear to work as an appetite suppressant."

> "My family doctor recommended that I try this diet as a safe alternative to prescription weight-loss medication. . . . Olive oil helps increase HDL (good) cholesterol. So even if it doesn't help you lose weight, it looks like it may have a few other advantages. I have used the oil for a week now. It has changed my appetite."

LEFTBLANC, who had posted extensively at Annie's Shangri-La Diet Blog, told calorielab.com readers that "I started this diet on 9/12 . . . I am 5′11″, and weighed 226 pounds. I now weigh 205 pounds" (November 23). CalorieLab replied, "Have you tried a more traditional calorie counting diet and not been able to stick to it? . . . I suspect that water or hot water in itself has an appetite suppressing effect simply by filling up your stomach," and went on to suggest a more traditional weight-loss plan ("avoid calorie-dense fast food, restaurant food, and packaged food"). Here is a bit of Leftblanc's long response:

"Why would I avoid restaurant food? I live in New York City, home to some of the greatest restaurants in the world. . . . This diet allows me to lose weight with a minimum of effort (and hunger). It's so much easier than counting calories. It's not like I didn't know a jelly doughnut had a lot of calories [during the seven years I weighed 226]; I ate it anyway."

STEPHEN M. joined the discussion:

"I can't say enough about the dramatic switch in the way I feel about food. I'm learning to think normally and act normally."

STARTING AT 240 pounds, he reported losing 15 pounds after 5 weeks. Yet another success:

"I'm a 52-year-old woman, 5 feet tall. I've been on the Shangri-La diet since September 17, 2005, and have gone from 163.50 pounds that day to 144.125 pounds today." [November 28. She lost nineteen pounds in eleven weeks.]

ALTHOUGH most comments have been positive, not all of them have been. On December 23, Imtiaz wrote:

"I have been trying the oil for about 8 days now and have not noticed any change in my appetite."

The blogosphere, so far, likes the diet—a lot. Maybe people are more likely to report success than failure, but this is a very promising beginning.

7

CHANGING THE REST OF THE WORLD

I didn't know any English at all when we came to the States. I knew hello, thank you, good-bye, *and for some obscure reason I knew the word* gluttony.

—KHALED HOSSEINI,
AUTHOR OF *The Kite Runner*

In the year 2001 so many physical problems will have been surmounted that . . . a woman will have a strong supple and splendid body all her life.

—1967 MEMO FROM DIANA VREELAND
(*Vogue* EDITOR IN CHIEF)

WHEN YOU understand what causes a problem, it becomes much easier to fix it. The reverse is true too: If you can efficiently fix a problem, it suggests you understand what caused it. Sugar water and flavorless oils will not only help people lose weight, they will help teach what causes obesity and how to prevent it.

This chapter is about prevention. Previous chapters have described solutions that are fairly easy and clear and that can begin tomorrow. This one is about solutions that require more effort, patience, persuasion, and thought.

A basic principle of problem solving is that the forces we can create, that we completely control, that we can turn on and off at will, are usually much weaker than preexisting forces we cannot turn on or off but merely point in a new direction. When a problem needs to be solved, I can do something whose sole purpose is to solve it (the direct approach) or I can modify what I was going to do anyway for other reasons (the preexisting force approach). If I need toothpaste, for example, I can take a trip to the store (direct) or I can wait until my other trips take me near a store (preexisting force). To get more exercise, I can go to a gym (direct) or I can start walking to work instead of riding the bus (preexisting force: I am already going to work). This chapter is about how two powerful preexisting forces—teachers and the food industry—can help prevent obesity in light of the ideas of this book. On my website (www.sethroberts.net), I say a little about what parents can do.

What Caused the Obesity Epidemic?

To do something about the obesity epidemic, it helps to know what caused it. In 1962, a large survey found that 13 percent of adult Americans were obese. In 1980, that percentage was 14 percent—essentially, the same. By 1993, however, it was 22 percent and by 2000 30 percent—a huge increase. Something very fattening began between 1980 and 1993.

What was it? Too little exercise, high-fat foods, soft drinks, and too-large portions are often blamed, but so are many other things. In *Food Fight* (2004), Kelly Brownell and Katherine Horgen point to several causes: television, video games, personal computers, eating away from home, snacking, and "the glorification of overeating." However, the evidence for most of these causes has been far from persuasive.

The sharp rise in obesity after 1980 is unlikely to be due to lack of exercise. First, there was no sharp drop in exercise after 1980. Time spent watching TV increased by 45 percent from 1965 to 1975, yet obesity increased little over that time; from 1975 to 1995, when obesity shot up, TV watching increased only a little. Second, if lack of exercise were a big cause of obesity, then getting more exercise should be a good way to lose weight. It is not. Unless you are completely sedentary to begin with, it is difficult to lose much weight through exercise alone. Oprah Winfrey provided unwitting proof of this when she started running half marathons. That's how fit she had had to become—to put it another way, how much exercise she had needed to do—in order to lose the weight she wanted to lose. In the 1950s, Americans were much thinner than now, but not because they were more active; if anything, they were less active. The President's Council on Physical Fitness was created in 1956 to address an alarming lack of fitness.

The obesity epidemic is unlikely to be due to a high-fat diet. In the 1950s, Americans were not eating low-fat diets, yet they were much thinner. Another reason to doubt that high-fat food is a common cause of obesity is that low-fat diets produce little weight loss. After a year, most people have lost only a few pounds.

The obesity epidemic is unlikely to be due to larger portions. From 1976 to 1996, calorie intake at breakfast, lunch, and dinner increased little, if at all; rather, there was a big increase in snacking. Restaurant portions have grown over the years, but I believe this is an effect of obesity rather than a cause of it. Restaurant portions did not physically grow during the three months I lost thirty-five pounds, but they came to appear huge—far more than I wanted to eat. Even after I stopped losing weight, they still appeared too large. My metabolism had slowed down. Likewise, when people gain weight their metabolism speeds up. They eat more and require larger portions to feel full.

So what *did* cause the obesity epidemic? The theory behind the Shangri-La diet (see Chapter 3, "A New Theory of Weight Control") is very clear. The most fattening foods, it says, are those that have all four of the following properties:

- A strong flavor.

- Quickly detected calories.

- Have been eaten many times.

- Have exactly the same flavor each time.

Might the consumption of such foods have greatly increased after 1980?

Junk food and fast food have these four properties; in fact, they have been engineered to have them. The table on page 128 gives some examples. Has consumption of these foods grown dramatically since 1980? The answer is yes. The economists Inas Rashad, at Georgia State University, and Michael Grossman, at the City University of New York Graduate Center, considered several possible causes for the obesity epidemic. "As much as two-thirds of the increase in adult obesity since 1980," they wrote, "can be explained by the rapid growth in the per capita number of fast-food restaurants and full-service restaurants, especially the former." Between 1960 and 1980, the per capita number of such restaurants grew slowly. After 1980, the number grew quickly. Figure 7, page 129, shows how closely the rise in obesity mirrored the rise in restaurants. From 1978 to 1996, calories eaten in sit-down restaurants doubled; calories eaten in fast-food restaurants tripled.

It's not just junk food and fast food. What I call ditto foods (foods that taste exactly the same each time) usually have these four properties as well. Ditto foods are found not only in restaurants and

THE FOUR PROPERTIES THAT MAKE FAST FOOD AND JUNK FOOD SO FATTENING

FOOD	STRONG FLAVOR FROM . . .	QUICKLY DETECTED CALORIES FROM . . .	UNIFORM FLAVOR FROM . . .	EATEN MANY TIMES BECAUSE . . .
Soft drink (Coke, Pepsi)	Secret ingredients	Glucose in high-fructose corn syrup	Mass production	Sold everywhere
Hamburger (McDonald's, Wendy's)	Ketchup, mustard, pickles, onions, secret sauce	Hamburger bun, french fries eaten at the same time	Standardized preparation, mass-produced ingredients	Sold everywhere
Pizza (Pizza Hut, Domino's)	Tomato sauce, toppings	White flour in crust	Standardized preparation, mass-produced ingredients	Sold everywhere
Doughnut (Krispy Kreme, Dunkin' Donuts)	Fillings, toppings	Sucrose, white flour	Mass production	Sold everywhere
Chocolate bar (Snickers, Mars)	Chocolate, flavorings	Sucrose	Mass production	Sold everywhere

vending machines. You eat them at home whenever you eat processed foods that need little or no preparation: breakfast cereals, microwaveable entrées, frozen pizza, crackers, orange juice from a carton, and cookies are just a few examples. The general name for these is *convenience foods*. They

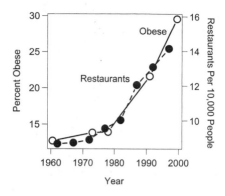

Figure 7. The growth of obesity in the United States from 1960 to 2000 closely parallels the growth in the number of restaurants.

are made in factories. They are supposed to taste exactly the same each time. In a 2003 paper, Harvard economists David Cutler, Edward Glaeser, and Jesse Shapiro, who knew nothing about my ideas, argued that the obesity epidemic was due to a great increase in the consumption of convenience foods (or, to put it another way, a great decrease in food preparation time) from 1978 to 1996. They had many types of evidence for this conclusion. For example, they found that the more reduction in food preparation time for various demographic categories (married women, single women, married men, single men) the greater the weight increase of persons in that category. Married women had the largest decrease in time spent preparing food, and gained the most weight.

Taken together, these ideas and facts give us good reason to think that the obesity epidemic is caused by eating too many foods with strong flavor-calorie associations. If this is correct, what should we do?

What Teachers Can Do

Obesity prevention naturally begins with children. After taking a tour of the Edible Schoolyard, a school garden in Berkeley, California, I asked an eighth-grader what she thought of it. She liked it, she said, because it had made her a better cook. "It's made me eat foods I didn't eat before. My mom's a good cook, though." Well, why didn't her mom's cooking have that effect? Because she refused to eat anything her mom made.

If a child's culinary mind is open only away from home, how can we take advantage of that? Dr. Antonia Demas, a food educator who founded the Food Studies Institute in upstate New York, may know better than anyone else how schools can persuade students to eat new foods.

In the late 1960s, Demas began to volunteer at a local Head Start center so that her infant son would be around older children. The food served there appalled her and she concentrated her volunteer efforts on improving it. Part of the problem was how to make the kids eat better foods. The solution, she noticed, was that the kids would eat anything they had helped make. So she taught them how to cook. Later, she volunteered in a second-grade classroom and continued to teach about food, connecting it with the teacher's lesson plan in creative and interesting ways. When the lesson topic was Native Americans, for example, she helped the students make traditional Iroquois corn soup, and compared flint corn to sweet corn. When the topic was archaeology, she told the students about the Bog People, ancient bodies discovered in the peat bogs of northern Europe. Because peat preserves soft tissues, researchers were able to determine their last meals, which were usually assortments of whole grains. So her students cooked a porridge of whole grains. Every two weeks Demas did another unit. "It stretched me in very creative ways," she said.

In the early 1990s, Demas decided to get a Ph.D. at nearby Cornell to document her curriculum development and make it available to other teachers. She conducted her dissertation research, a simple experiment, at a local elementary school. Half of the school's teachers agreed to let her teach units in their classes. They were the treatment group. The remaining twelve classes, taught by other teachers, did not receive Demas's curriculum. They were the control group.

She taught sixteen different lessons, with sixteen different foods, in each of the twelve treatment classes. For a lesson on India, the students made curry, a mixture of spices, sweet potatoes, carrots, and lots of other vegetables, with brown rice on the side. For a lesson on North Africa, the food was a stew of chickpeas, beans, tomatoes, zucchini, and other vegetables, with whole wheat couscous. From the point of view of obesity prevention all of these foods were excellent. Their flavors were unfamiliar, they contained no source of quickly detected calories, they were homemade and complex, so the flavor would vary quite a bit each time they were made, and they were not widely available.

After she had given a particular lesson in all twelve treatment classrooms, the food cooked at that lesson was served as a side dish for lunch in the cafeteria. It was not optional: It was put on every child's tray. After lunch, each side-dish container was weighed to determine how much of the food had been eaten.

The main result was very clear. Children in the treatment classes usually ate most or all of the side dish. Children in the control classes almost always ate none of it.

The lessons had other effects. As the year progressed, children in the treatment classes ate more and more of the lesson foods at lunchtime. They became more and more used to trying the new foods they had cooked. From conversations that Demas overheard, she learned that it had become cool to eat as many different foods as possible and to eat unusual foods.

The effects went beyond the school cafeteria. The kids took the recipes home and made them for their families. They told their parents about the virtues of the ingredients. They got excited about cooking. Demas ran into parents at the supermarket. "I can't believe it," the parent would say. "My kid wants to eat this food, wants me to buy ingredients so she can prepare it." They would never have believed that their kids would want to eat any of this food, much less want to prepare it.

After receiving her Ph.D. in 1995, Demas helped start similar teaching programs in Santa Fe, New Mexico, and Rochester, New York. Today, her work is used in more than four hundred schools. In Santa Fe, the program, called Cooking with Kids, has grown from two schools to ten schools, with about four thousand students participating. Demas continues her research. In South Bend, Indiana, she recently completed a study in which she was able to learn what the parents of children in her program bought at the supermarket. Purchases of the more unusual foods, such as collard greens, escarole, and bulgur wheat, went way up, and the increases lasted at least six months after the program ended. Three-quarters of the children in her program lost weight. It's an excellent start.

Another way to improve what children eat is suggested by a story in *Totto-Chan* (1981), a memoir by Tetsuko Kuroyanagi, a TV star in Japan, of her elementary-school days. Kuroyanagi attended a small private school in Tokyo during World War II. On Sports Day, a Japanese national holiday, schools everywhere have athletic competitions. One of many wonderful and special things about Kuroyanagi's school was that the Sports Day prizes were vegetables: "First Prize might be a giant radish; Second Prize, two burdock roots; Third Prize, a bundle of spinach," wrote Kuroyanagi. The children grumbled about these prizes, so the headmaster spoke to them. "Get your mothers to cook them for dinner tonight. They're vegetables you earned yourselves. You have provided food for your families by your own efforts. How's that? I bet it tastes good!" Kuroyanagi added, "He was right." It's not just an interesting idea; it's an interesting idea that worked.

What the Food Industry Can Do

In the battle against obesity, big food companies are not the enemy, as many public health advocates seem to think. This belief is counterproductive and unfair. When Americans believed that fat caused obesity, food companies made many low-fat products. When Americans believed that carbohydrates caused obesity, companies made many low-carb products. If these products had worked better, food companies would have made more of them.

If the Shangri-La diet and the theory behind it have merit, what new products and services might we expect from the food industry, besides the obvious (bottled sugar water and tote-sized ELOO)?

- *More consumer control of flavor.* For example, frozen pizza with ten optional toppings, to be added in creative combinations by the chef— the person who heats it up. The more novel the flavor combinations, the less fattening the food would be. At a movie theater I attended recently, you could flavor your popcorn using twelve different shakers, with flavors such as apple cinnamon, ranch, and chocolate marshmallow.

- *Lots of new flavors.* Mango-mint soda, anyone? A flavor-of-the-month program created by soft drink companies might work. The new flavors wouldn't be available long enough to become familiar.

- *More slowly digested foods.* This means foods with a lower glycemic index, as discussed in Chapter 6, "Extra Credit: Six More Ways to Lose Weight." A first step is adding a food's glycemic index to the mandatory nutritional information on the package. Some Australian food manufacturers put something called the GI Symbol (www.gisymbol.com.au) on food labels, along with the food's glycemic index. Cargill, a huge American ingredients company, recently introduced two new sweeteners (one liquid, one powder) whose key property is that they are slowly digested. Because these sweeteners are caloric, they can be used to make sugar water for the Shangri-La diet.

- *Low-flavor foods.* "Half the flavor, all the calories" sounds more sarcastic than appetizing. But low-salt foods are found in every supermarket.

Foods with less added flavor than usual may be possible as well, perhaps under the name *delicate-flavor foods*. Delicately flavored foods, even when eaten many times, will raise the set point less than strongly flavored foods.

- *Emphasis on qualities other than flavor.* Foods with weaker flavor-calorie associations taste less good—there is no avoiding this. But Food A may have a weaker flavor-calorie association than Food B, yet still be as pleasant as Food B if Food A is superior to Food B in other ways that bring us pleasure, such as appearance and texture. Sushi is very popular, for instance, yet it usually has a weak flavor. Excellent appearance and texture compensate for the weak flavor. A particularly good take-out pizza store near my house offers only one topping per day. Every day, the topping changes. They reap little benefit from flavor-calorie associations, but their pizza is wildly popular because of its originality, great appearance, great texture, and a certain something that comes from using high-end ingredients.

- *Promote connoisseurship.* Food connoisseurs avoid ditto foods—exactly the foods that my theory says you should avoid. They search out, purchase, eat, and even glorify foods with unusual and subtle flavors—exactly the foods my theory says you should eat. Inevitably these foods are made in small batches and cannot become very familiar. A culture of food connoisseurship may be the main reason that the French are less obese than Americans.

- *Foods that intentionally vary in flavor.* During that fateful trip to Paris (see Chapter 2, "The Case of the Missing Appetite"), I drank ordinary soft drinks and lost weight. They caused weight loss because their flavors were unfamiliar. Could a soda be made whose flavor would *always* be unfamiliar? Yes, if the flavor varied enough from one serving to the next. To produce such a soda would require a new kind of manufacturing. Food companies (and other manufacturers) work hard to ensure that their products are always the same. Quality control in manufacturing means minimizing variation. The goal of this new kind of manufacturing would be to *introduce* variation in a controlled way—enough so that the soda is far less fattening, but not so much that consumers are confused. It is probably impossible to make each bottle different from every other bottle, but the goal would be to introduce enough variation so that the flavor would never become familiar. If the variation were large enough, drinking this newfangled soda would help you lose weight, just as I lost weight in Paris. It would be better than plain sugar water because you could drink it at meals. If you drink *unflavored* sugar water at a meal, it will simply strengthen the flavor-calorie associations of the flavors of the rest of the meal. *Flavored* sugar water will not have this effect. The flavor of the sugar water will interfere with the association of the flavors of other foods and the sugar-water calories.

In recent years, big food companies have clearly been interested in making their product lines healthier. Coca-Cola bought Odwalla, a manufacturer of fruit juices, for exactly that reason. McDonald's introduced more salad variety and put fresh fruit on their menu. What I hope will interest food company executives is the idea that *you can make a weight-loss version of Coke.* This is completely new. It would require substantial innovations in manufacturing, but the potential market for this product and the other products and services I have described is enormous.

The Antidote to Civilization

Club Med, the resort chain, used to call itself "the antidote to civilization"—a brilliant and revealing slogan. It revealed two things: A substantial fraction of the target audience (people rich enough to afford Club Med) was (a) slightly miserable (thus needing an "antidote") and (b) convinced that civilization was the source of their discontent. Club Med offered a vaguely pre-civilized life—for example, outdoor activities, no money—for a week or two.

The obesity epidemic is clearly a by-product of civilization. We don't just have plenty of food; we also have enough money to pay for considerable processing of that food. Proposed solutions to the obesity epidemic have often had a Club Med–like flavor: Outlaw television. Make exercise mandatory. No foods introduced since 1950. These solutions are appealing, alas, for the same reason Club Med is appealing: We believe in our hearts that something is wrong with civilization.

These views are not wrong, exactly, but they are doughnut truths. Something crucial is missing. The urban theorist and author Jane Jacobs had a great way of putting it. In discussing what to do about pollution, she said the problem is not too much this or too little that; the problem is the undone work— by which she meant the intricate, time-consuming development of new ideas and new products and services based on those ideas. The antidote to civilization, Jacobs would say, is more civilization.

A diet book is a low form of civilization. In this chapter, I have indicated what some higher forms might be, including new school curricula and new food products. They are only the beginning. When creative and resourceful people have the right ideas about the causes of obesity, they will begin to change our world in many ways that make it much harder to become obese.

Appendix

THE SCIENCE BEHIND THE THEORY BEHIND THE DIET

"Am I the only one who thinks this diet might be an enormous hoax perpetrated by the *Freakonomics* guys?" posted someone on a blog about the Shangri-La diet. "I hardly believe it myself," someone replied—someone for whom it was working. They weren't the only ones. After *Good Morning America* ran a piece about it, Diane Sawyer's first words were: "Jaws are dropping around the studio." One reason the diet is so surprising is that it is based on science that most people—including, unfortunately, most obesity researchers—are unaware of.

I would like to change that. You don't need to know about the science to do the diet; that's why this is an appendix. But for those who are interested, here's a brief explanation of the scientific basis for the diet, especially the work of the three scientists—Michel Cabanac, Anthony Sclafani, and Israel Ramirez—who influenced me the most.

Physiology Meets Psychology

The theory behind the Shangri-La diet is based on research in two areas that are usually separate: weight control and associative learning. Most weight control researchers know little about associative learning, and most associative learning researchers know little about weight control. The two topics are studied in different university departments: weight control in physiology, associative learning in psychology.

A central concept in physiology is *homeostasis:* the maintenance of constant conditions. Throughout our bodies, homeostasis is happening in hundreds of ways. Sweating when you are hot and shivering when you are cold are ways your brain keeps your body temperature constant. The oil on your skin is another example. Washing your face causes your oil glands to become more active in order to restore the oil you washed away. The concentrations of many substances in your blood, including oxygen and glucose (blood sugar), are kept constant in various ways.

Around 1950, a London researcher named G. Kennedy made observations about the weight of rats that suggested that body fat too was homeostatically regulated. The rats were fed rat chow mixed with water. Kennedy varied how much water was mixed with the chow. When the amount of water was doubled, thus cutting the density of calories in half, for a few days the rats ate fewer calories than usual. As a result, they lost weight. A few days after that, however, they started eating more calories than usual, enough to regain the lost weight. Subsequently, they ate enough each day to stay at their pre-dilution weight. Their weight remained quite constant even when their food changed a lot, just as a thermostat-controlled heating-and-cooling system keeps a room's temperature roughly the same even when the outside temperature changes. Kennedy proposed that a thermostat-like system—in other words, a system with a set point—controls our weight.

Kennedy's proposal was supported by the discovery of the hormone leptin in 1994. In order to regulate the amount of body fat, the brain must be able to know how much body fat you have, just as a thermostat needs a built-in thermometer to keep track of the room temperature. Leptin serves as the brain's body-fat thermometer: The concentration of leptin in your blood tells your brain how much fat is in your body. Leptin is produced by fat cells. When your body fat goes up, so does the amount of leptin in your blood. When your body fat goes down, leptin goes down.

Associative learning is as central to psychology as homeostasis is to physiology. One type of associative learning is Pavlovian conditioning, discovered by Ivan Pavlov, the Russian physiologist. In laboratory experiments, Pavlov found that if he rang a bell for two minutes and then gave a dog food, the dog quickly learned to associate the sound of the bell with arrival of the food. After several of these bell-food pairings, ringing the bell would cause the dog to salivate in anticipation of receiving food.

The generalizations that Pavlov discovered by studying bells, food, and salivation turned out to predict what happens in many other situations. They have helped us understand fear, hunger, food aversions, drug tolerance, drug addiction, sexual arousal, and even visual aftereffects. My graduate training was close to this area of psychology.

Kennedy's set point theory of weight control and Pavlov's learning experiments are well known. They were the starting points for the science that led to my theory.

Michel Cabanac: The University of Cold Water

Dr. Michel Cabanac is a professor of physiology at Laval University, in Quebec. His first research project, as a medical student in Lyon, France, was about thermoregulation in dogs. After graduation, in 1958, he went to Paris, where his boss assigned him to study thermoregulation in humans. The research involved subjects sitting in a tub of hot water. One day Cabanac himself served as a subject. The hot water made him very warm. Cleaning the equipment afterward, he got some cold water on his hands and he noticed it felt good. "To me this was

Newton's apple," he said, referring to the story that a falling apple inspired Newton's theory of gravity. He suddenly had an idea about why we feel pleasure and pain. Part of what makes a temperature feel pleasant or unpleasant, he realized, was a *difference:* the difference between the body's set point temperature (the temperature the system tries to maintain) and the body's actual (core) temperature. If your core temperature is *more* than your set point, cold water feels pleasant. That was Cabanac's situation: Sitting in the hot water had raised his core temperature above his set point. But if your core temperature is *less* than your set point, cold water feels unpleasant. Because we seek and continue pleasant experiences and avoid or end unpleasant ones, these hedonic changes help us regulate our body temperature.

Cabanac wanted to test his idea about pleasure in other domains. Food is another source of pleasure. Do changes in how pleasant we find food help regulate our weight? He began to study what controls how pleasant we find a sip of sugar water. For years, he got nowhere; nothing he tried changed how his subjects responded. He did find that if subjects were given glucose in water through a tube into their stomach, sips of sugar water became less pleasant. This was a whittled-down laboratory version of what happens during a meal: Calories go into your stomach, your body senses the calories, food becomes less pleasant (and when it reaches "not pleasant," you stop eating). Just as the pleasantness of cold water depends on the difference between set point temperature and core temperature, Cabanac believed that the pleasantness of sweet water would depend on the difference between body-weight set point and actual weight.

To test this prediction, he did an experiment in which subjects lost eight pounds by eating less of their usual food. This was meant to lower their actual weight below their set point. He was one of the subjects. He told me, "It was torture. You dream you are breaking the fast and ruining the experiment." At the lower weight, glucose water sent directly into the stomach through a tube no longer reduced how pleasant sips of sweet water tasted. A force that pushes people to stop eating—the food stops tasting good—was no longer present. Cabanac concluded that when your weight is below your set point, it takes more food to feel full. Implicit in this was the prediction that when your weight is *above* your set point, it will take *less* food to feel full.

Cabanac's experiment came to life for me when countless Shangri-La dieters spoke of needing much less food to feel full. "This is the first time I have ever left food on a plate at a meal," wrote one. "I'm able to feel full after eating about half of what I normally eat," wrote another. I had had the same experience. These comments were an excellent sign that the Shangri-La diet works as I theorized: It lowers your set point.

Cabanac did another experiment to see if the "laws" of temperature regulation applied to weight regulation. In temperature regulation, skin temperature affects the set point. Warming the skin lowers the body temperature set point; cooling the skin raises the set point. "This anticipates future threat," said Cabanac. The key idea is that the set point is sensitive to prevailing conditions in the outside world.

To see if something similar happened with weight, Cabanac and a colleague did an experiment in which subjects got all their calories from what Cabanac called "a very flat food," a bland liquid diet. The subjects, one of whom was Cabanac, could eat as much of the liquid diet as they wanted, but they still lost weight, as Cabanac had predicted. In contrast to calorie restriction ("torture"), this way of losing weight was "painless," said Cabanac. "The subjects, including myself, lost and lost and lost weight and did not suffer. Without feeling hungry—never." The experiment continued until they had lost as much weight as the subjects in the earlier calorie-restriction experiment. Then, while the subjects were at their lower weight, the glucose-loading test was repeated. This time the results were perfectly normal: The glucose load in the stomach made sips of the sweet water taste less pleasant. Cabanac's explanation is that in this case the weight loss did not change the results because set point and actual weight stayed close. When you lose weight by eating bland food (easy), your set point goes down. When you lose weight by calorie restriction (hard), your set point doesn't go down.

That there are two quite different ways of losing weight—with and without set point reduction—is a very important idea.

The bland food experiment also impressed me because it demonstrated with human subjects that your set point depends on what you eat. Unfortunately, Cabanac's work didn't receive the attention it deserved. When I asked him what the rest of the world made of it, he said he didn't think it had been cited at all in other professional publications. He checked, however, and found that it had been cited twenty times since publication in 1976—not much, considering the vast interest in weight loss.

Around the same time as the bland food experiment, a student in Cabanac's lab named Marc Fantino, who is now a medical school professor in Dijon, France, did a similar but more extreme experiment, in which four subjects got all of their nutrition via a tube through the nose into the stomach—nutrition without any flavor at all, in other words. They could consume as much as they wanted but lost weight quickly, quite a bit faster than the subjects in the bland-food experiment, even though the food was the same. This suggested to me that flavor raised the set point. Without any flavor, the set point went down quickly.

Surely, I thought, some flavors were more potent than others. What did you need to know about a flavor to predict *how much* it would increase the set point? Cabanac's and Fantino's research raised this question but did not help answer it.

Anthony Sclafani: Why We Like Spinach

Dr. Anthony Sclafani is a professor of psychology at Brooklyn College, a branch of the City University of New York. In the 1970s, he was looking for an animal model of obesity. It is surprisingly hard to make normal rats fat. At the time, the usual way of making rats fat was to add fat to their chow by mixing in a solid shortening, such as Crisco. This produced obesity, but slowly. Maybe if the food tasted better, they would get fat more quickly, reasoned Sclafani. He sent one of his graduate students to the supermarket and had him bring back fattening foods such as sweetened condensed milk, chocolate-chip cookies, salami, cheese, bananas, marshmallows, milk chocolate, and peanut butter.

When young, still-growing rats were given these foods in addition to rat chow, they gained weight more than twice as fast as when given only rat chow, and much faster than rats given a high-fat diet. This suggested that supermarket food was quite fattening compared to rat chow, and that it was not just its high fat content that made it fattening. This research was published in the same year (1976) and journal (*Physiology & Behavior*) as Cabanac's bland-food experiment, separated by just a few hundred pages. Both experiments—rat (Sclafani), human (Cabanac), weight gain (Sclafani), weight loss (Cabanac)—suggested to me that the flavor of food controls the set point. Good-tasting food raises the set point; not-so-good-tasting food lowers it.

Ten years later, Sclafani was still studying food intake. By accident, he had discovered that rats have a remarkable appetite for a partially digested starch called Polycose. To humans this is a bland source of calories; if you add it to orange juice, it doesn't change the flavor. But rats loved it. This attractiveness had a curious quality: It increased over days. For example, rats initially preferred sugar water to Polycose water, but over a period of several days switched their preference to the Polycose solution. This suggested to Sclafani that Polycose had powerful effects *after* ingestion that caused its taste to become very attractive. The notion that flavors become better tasting when they are associated with calories or nutrients that are detected by the digestive system had been kicking around since the 1960s. But there had been only a few demonstrations of such learning and in those cases the learning had been weak.

Maybe, thought Sclafani, the question—*Does flavor–calorie associative learning really exist?*—was worth revisiting. Sclafani and a colleague set up an apparatus that would inject either Polycose water or plain water directly into a rat's stomach whenever it drank. The experiment used two flavors of Kool-Aid. When a rat drank water with Flavor 1, it got Polycose water injected into its stomach. When it drank water with Flavor 2, it got plain water injected into its stomach. In contrast to the weak effects of earlier research, this procedure produced a huge preference for water with Flavor 1 when the rat was given a choice between the two flavors. Even after the Polycose injections were stopped and both Kool-Aid flavors were followed by injections of plain water, the preference persisted for days.

Sclafani hadn't discovered flavor-calorie learning; earlier researchers had done that. What he *had* done was discover its importance, its power, and how to study it. In the following years, Sclafani and his colleagues did hundreds of experiments about flavor-calorie learning. They made it real. By the time I started theorizing about weight control, it was so firmly established that I took it for granted.

Israel Ramirez: Connecting Associative Learning and Weight Control

When Dr. Israel Ramirez worked at the Monell Chemical Senses Institute, in Philadelphia (1982–1997), he did one brilliant experiment after another. Psychology and physiology research is intensely empirical. Everything revolves around data, usually from experiments. Compared to other scientists who study food intake, Cabanac is a great theorist whose experiments deftly support his theoretical ideas, and Sclafani is a great empiricist whose experiments make a rich pointillist picture of an empirical generalization. Ramirez was a

Shakespearean court jester type of scientist whose experiments obliquely spoke deep truths.

On the face of it, Ramirez was a scientist whose specialty was doing experiments with hard-to-explain results. This is a difficult position for a scientist. Puzzling results are the most enlightening, or at least they can be, but it may take quite a while to figure out the explanation, and in the meantime the value of your work is unclear. Ramirez singlehandedly gave the whole field of weight control a big push forward, but it was not obvious at the time.

Ramirez is now a software consultant and developer at PC Helps Support, Bala Cynwd, Pennsylvania. He did so much great work at Monell that when I interviewed him in 2005 he did not remember an outstanding review paper he had written twenty years earlier about whether sugar causes obesity. "It is widely believed," the paper began, "that consumption of sucrose may predispose human beings to obesity." Ramirez concluded, however, that "animal [rat] studies do not support [this] idea." He pointed out that sugar has a much different effect on weight when it is eaten "wet" (dissolved in water) than when eaten dry. This is not consistent with the simple idea that sugar is fattening. Because rats and humans are quite similar in many dietary ways, this was powerful evidence against the conventional view.

After Sclafani commented that rats given bread in addition to their regular chow became obese, Ramirez decided to do a simple experiment. He compared two groups of rats given bread as their only source of calories. One group got ordinary bread mix modified so that it was nutritionally complete. The other group got the same mix in the form of actual bread, which was made by adding water to the mix and baking it. Thus the two groups were offered the same nutrients, the same micronutrients, the same proportions of fat, carbohydrate, and protein. After several weeks, the rats given cooked bread weighed substantially more than the rats given bread mix. The experiment is so simple and easy that a seventh-grader could do it, yet it shows that something important is missing from conventional weight-control ideas. "It was an ugly sort of thing," he told me. (In fact, it was beautifully simple, both in thought and execution. By "ugly" Ramirez meant it was hard to say exactly how the cooked bread differed from the uncooked bread.) When he told colleagues about it, "it evoked a bit of laughter." He didn't publish it.

He did think about it, though. One difference between the bread mix and the bread was the water added to make the bread. So Ramirez did several experiments that measured the effect of adding water to dry rat chow. They showed that water was fattening—very fattening! Young rats given wet food gained more weight than rats given dry food, even though both groups had water available from a water bottle. The effect was huge: The right amount of water could *double* the rats' weight gain. This contradicts everything the average American has been told about weight control. Dieters are always told to drink lots of water, because water has no calories, no fat, no carbohydrate, no sugar, no anything. When I tell people this result they are usually dumbfounded. Ramirez himself was unsure how to explain it. My theory, however, explains this astonishing result because it is likely that moistening the chow both increased its flavor and speeded up its digestion, thereby leading to stronger flavor-calorie associations.

Sclafani's flavor-calorie learning experiments demonstrated something that many others had believed but had been unable to show. Cabanac's experiments were beautiful demonstrations that exposed a hidden logic already known to Cabanac. Ramirez's experiments, on the other hand, usually exposed everyone's *lack* of understanding, including his own.

One set of Ramirez's experiments went further. Like so many important discoveries, it began with a kind of accident. Along the lines of the bread experiment, Ramirez was wondering how to cause "overeating" without changing macronutrient (fat/protein/carbohydrate) composition. Farmers had tried adding saccharin to livestock feed in order to fatten their animals more quickly. Maybe the saccharin would make the food taste better so the animals would eat more of it. As far as Ramirez knew, this had always failed. But maybe it was worth another try.

The experimental design was simple: He used

two groups of rats. Both groups were given a liquid diet (the diet needed to be liquid so that the saccharin could be added). One group got the liquid diet with saccharin; the other group got the liquid diet without saccharin. The first two experiments gave inconsistent results. In one Ramirez got an effect (the rats given saccharin ate more and gained more weight), in the other he didn't. "[A colleague] was looking at my results," Ramirez said. "He thought it was silly: Half were successful, half weren't."

Ramirez assumed that the reason for the inconsistent results was that some rats naturally liked saccharin and some did not. If he could sort the rats into those two groups—those that liked saccharin and those that didn't—the results should become strong and clear. The rats that liked saccharin would gain weight, and the ones that didn't like it would not. So he did an experiment in which he measured how much each rat liked saccharin before going on to measure the effect of saccharin on each rat's weight.

This experiment had a curious result: Saccharin had no effect. The weights of the two groups did not differ. Yet the only difference between this experiment and an earlier experiment where saccharin *did* have an effect was the saccharin-preference test at the beginning. Ramirez had assumed that the preference test itself would not affect the rats' weight. Preference tests are harmless, right? If someone asks you how much you like chocolate, surely that does not make chocolate any less fattening. If you fill out a three-page survey about hot dogs, surely that does not make the hot dogs you eat less fattening. The saccharin preference test had consisted of giving rats a bottle of saccharin-flavored water in their home cage (in addition to plain water) for four days. The rats that drank the most saccharin-flavored water were assumed to like saccharin the most. Surely such an innocuous experience would not affect the rats' weight. But it did. A new experiment, in which some rats were given the preference test and others were not, showed this conclusively.

One way to think about the results was this: Only if the saccharin was *new* would adding it to the liquid diet make that diet more fattening. If the saccharin was familiar, it did not make the liquid diet more fattening. Ramirez looked at the earlier experiment that had failed to find an effect of saccharin. In that experiment, the rats had gotten the liquid diet for one week before the saccharin was added. This suggested that the *liquid diet* must also be new when it is combined with saccharin for the saccharin to be effective. All in all, the experiments suggested that *experience* with a food affected how fattening it was. That is one of the key ideas of my weight control theory. At the end of the scientific paper about these results, Ramirez wrote that "the present report provides the first evidence that learning may be an important factor in dietary hyperphagia [overeating]."

Indeed it did. This was a radical new idea. Apparently no one who read the paper knew what to make of it. It was rarely cited. "You picked up on it," Ramirez told me in 2005. "No one else did."

Because of my graduate training in psychology, I knew a lot about Pavlovian conditioning. That the saccharin and the liquid diet both had to be new to the rats in order to get the effect immediately suggested to me that Pavlovian conditioning was involved; more specifically, it suggested that the effect was due to a *learned association* between the flavor of the saccharin and the calories of the liquid diet. Because of Sclafani's work, I took it for granted that such learning happened. Because of Cabanac's work, I assumed that anything that increased weight did so by raising the set point. Cabanac and Sclafani had persuasively demonstrated that what you eat, especially its flavor, can influence your body-weight set point, so it was easy to believe that flavor-calorie associations affected the set point. There was a little more to my new theory than that, but not much.

For more about the science behind the theory, see www.sethroberts.net/articles/whatmakesfood fattening.pdf.

ACKNOWLEDGMENTS

IF MY Croatian friend Jasmina Kos had not invited me to visit her, causing me to spend a week in Paris . . . thanks, Jasmina. Carl Willat has been endlessly helpful and encouraging, including the curious suggestion that this book be circle shaped and titled *You Look Like This*. "Help it stand out," he said.

I am grateful to the many friends who tried my weight-loss methods and told their friends about them. Their experiences were the first signs that these ideas could help many people. My students have been a cheerful and inquisitive audience and have had a way of testing my ideas without telling me, which I found quite complimentary.

For help with the research behind this book, I want to thank Janessa Karawan, who continued to assist me even after she got a full-time job because she thought it was such an interesting project, Katie Kelly, who helped in many ways, and my mother, Justine Roberts (a medical librarian). My mom, who knew all about database searches long before Google—when they were called *queries*—did hundreds of them to help me out.

I thank Margaret Adamek, Elizabeth Capaldi, David Cutler, William Jacobs, Frances Jalet-Miller, Naomi Katz, Inas Rashad (who also helped with Figure 7), Paul Rozin, and Norman Temple for speaking with me. Michel Cabanac, Antonia Demas, Israel Ramirez, and Anthony Sclafani (who also gave me a tour of his lab) each spent several hours answering my questions. In the Appendix I try to explain how important the work of Cabanac, Ramirez, and Sclafani has been to my thinking. Israel Ramirez talked to me at length ten years ago, too. My theory of weight control was inspired by one of the twenty-odd reprints of his papers that he sent me back then.

That was before open access (free availability of research via the Web). The combination of open access and blogs did wonders for this book. Stevan Harnad has not only pushed for open access for many years; he founded *Behavioral and Brain Sciences,* where the scientific article behind this book was published, built it into a highly cited open access journal, and was the editor who accepted my article. I am very grateful to Andrew Gelman, a longtime friend, who wrote about my work at www.stat.columbia.edu/~gelman/blog. Open access meant readers of his blog could read my article and see for themselves. His comments drew the attention of Alex Tabarrok at the Marginal Revolution (www.marginalrevolution.com), who wrote the most favorable notice my work has ever received.

Stephen Dubner and Steven Levitt, the authors of *Freakonomics,* learned about my work via Marginal Revolution, and drew it to the attention of the book industry, not to mention the general public, via a column in *The New York Times.* Not only did they try my ideas themselves, they invited me to guest-blog at www.freakonomics.com. That led Ann Hendricks to set up a blog where people trying the Shangri-La diet—the bootleg version—could swap stories. Their stories and enthusiasm made writing this book much easier, as I mentioned in the Introduction.

My agent, Suzanne Gluck, as she so often does, did a great job of generating interest among publishers; whenever something good happens related to this book, I call it "the Gluck effect." Laura Bellotti helped me prepare a proposal and sample chapters that Suzanne had very little quarrel with.

"Everyone needs an editor," says a friend of mine. I need an editor more than most—thank goodness Marian Lizzi, my editor at Putnam, was there for me. When I was unsure about what to do—and this happened a lot—I would phone Marian and ask. I'm a little amazed how often I agreed with her suggestions. Helping me write the book, Sheila Buff provided a good sounding board, much-needed health expertise, and cogent advice.

"The diet book with a Ph.D.," Marian has wittily called it. My Ph.D. is in experimental psychology, and in several ways this is the sort of book an experimental psychologist would write (e.g., taking experiments with rats seriously). I have learned more experimental psychology from Saul Sternberg, a research scientist at Bell Labs and a professor at the University of Pennsylvania, than from anyone else. He has been incredibly supportive throughout my academic career. When I was a graduate student, Saul invited me to give a talk at Bell Labs. Afterward, we had dinner at his house. There was a graph of some data on the refrigerator. "What's this?" I asked. "The force of gravity," he said. It was a graph of his weight.

In the afterword to *Exploratory Data Analysis* (1977), a great statistics book, John Tukey wrote that he hadn't mentioned computers in the main text but their shadow fell on every page. This book is dedicated to animal-learning researchers because my debt to them is no less than Tukey's to computers. They built up a body of work, thousands of experiments about associative learning and how to study it, without which this book would never have been possible.

NOTES

Abbreviations

Annie's blog: www.blogger.com/comment.g?blogID
=16962289&postID=112729758775514780

CalorieLab blog: calorielab.com/news/2005/09/21/
seth-roberts-shangri-la-diet-in-detail

Epigraph

ix "Curiously enough, the immense dinner . . . hungrier than usual": Nancy Mitford, *Love in a Cold
Climate* (New York: Modern Library, 1994), 339.

Introduction

2   when I wrote for *Spy* magazine: Seth Roberts,
"Lab Rat: What AIDS Researcher Dr. Robert
Gallo Did in Pursuit of the Nobel Prize, and What

He Didn't Do in Pursuit of a Cure for AIDS," *Spy*, June 1990, 70–79. Available at www.virusmyth. net/aids/data/srlabrat.htm accessed December 15, 2005.

3 "The common aim of all science . . . the gradual removal of prejudices": Niels Bohr, *Atomic Physics and Human Knowledge* (New York: John Wiley Science Editions, 1961), p. 31.

Chapter 1. Why a Calorie Is Not a Calorie

5 One of the guys said to the other . . . a one-pound box of candy and gain 10 pounds": Mary Kate Norton, "Men Are Pigs," *The Daily Californian,* July 25, 2000, 3.

5 the term *doughnut truth* to mean "only the truth, and the whole truth, with a hole in the truth": Vladimir Nabokov, *Ada* (New York: McGraw-Hill, 1969), 154.

6 Everything should be about portion size: Marion Nestle comment during the "Table for Twelve," segment of *On the Media* (WNYC), April 22, 2005. Transcript at www.onthemedia.org/transcripts/ transcripts__042205__food.html accessed January 5, 2005.

17 He later wrote it tasted "like medicine": Gaku Homma, *The Folk Art of Japanese Country Cooking* (Berkeley, Calif.: North Atlantic Books, 1991), 21.

17 "First put off by the leaves' flavor, after repeated exposure I grew to anticipate their taste":

Jonathan Kauffman, "A Star Is Stewed," *East Bay Express*, October 6, 2004. At www.eastbayexpress.com/Issues/2004-10-06/dining/food__print.html accessed December 9, 2005.

19 Research has shown that the brain treats sweetness differently from other flavors: Elizabeth D. Capaldi, "Conditioned Food Preferences," in Elizabeth D. Capaldi, ed., *Why We Eat What We Eat: The Psychology of Eating* (Washington, D.C.: American Psychological Association, 1996).

Chapter 2. The Case of the Missing Appetite

21 This new, $3 billion-a-year industry was aimed squarely at . . . never works: Margaret Webb Pressler, "Low-Carb Fad Fades, and Atkins Is Big Loser," *The Washington Post*, August 2, 2005, A01.

26 There was no precedent anywhere . . . causing so much weight loss: For more about my weight-loss self-experimentation, see Seth Roberts, "Self-experimentation as a Source of New Ideas: Ten Examples About Sleep, Mood, Health, and Weight," *Behavioral and Brain Sciences* 27 (2) (April 2004): 227–288. Available at repositories.cdlib.org/postprints/117.

29 "There is something unpleasant or aversive about sweetness when food deprivation is high" . . . based on her research: Elizabeth D. Capaldi, "Conditioned Food Preferences," in Elizabeth D. Capaldi, ed., *Why We Eat What We Eat: The Psychology of Eating* (Washington,

D.C.: American Psychological Association, 1996).
Quotation from p. 67.

31 Olive oil is a staple of the Mediterranean diet,
eaten by groups of people . . . have low rates of
heart disease (and little obesity): Walter C.
Willett et al. "Mediterranean Diet Pyramid: A
Cultural Model for Healthy Eating," *American
Journal of Clinical Nutrition* 61, Suppl. 6 (June
1995): 1402S–1406S. Chapter 4 of *Eat, Drink, and
Be Healthy: The Harvard Medical School Guide
to Healthy Eating* (New York: Simon & Schuster,
2002), by Walter Willett, describes other reasons
to think olive oil is healthy.

32 My metabolism had slowed down: Experiments
with rats and humans have shown that your
metabolism slows down. For example, see Jules
Hirsch, Lisa C. Hudgins, Rudolph L. Leibel, and
Michael Rosenbaum, "Diet Composition and
Energy Balance in Humans," *American Journal
of Clinical Nutrition* 67, Suppl. 3 (1998):
551S–555S.

33 According to *New Yorker* writer Malcolm
Gladwell, diet books "have an unspoken set of
narrative rules and conventions . . . the radical
truth that inspired his diet": Malcolm Gladwell,
"The Pima Paradox," *The New Yorker,* February
2, 1998. Available at www.gladwell.com/1998/
1998_02_02_a_pima.htm accessed January 27,
2006.

35 "Weight loss is not for the fainthearted," said
Dr. Thomas Wadden . . . in 2005: Gina Kolata,

"Diet and Lose Weight? Scientists Say 'Prove It!,' " *The New York Times,* January 4, 2005.

Chapter 4. How to Do the Shangri-La Diet

54 Secretly, I suspected the answer to weight issues would be something ridiculously simple, but this is almost too much to hope for: Emily Jones, "Another Venture into La La Land," *Starkville Daily News,* November 16, 2005. At http://starkvilledailynews.com/articles/2005/11 /16/news/lifestyles/lifestyles02 accessed November 21, 2005.

54 It appealed to my essential laziness: http:// CalorieLab blog/#comment-743 (Leftblanc, posted November 25, 2005) accessed November 25, 2005.

59 Another reason I chose fructose instead of sucrose . . . when fructose is the source of the calories: Karen Ackroff, Khalid Touzani, Tatanisha K. Peets, and Anthony Sclafani, "Flavor preferences conditioned by intragastric fructose and glucose: Differences in reinforcement potency," *Physiology & Behavior* 72 (5) (April 2001): 691–703.

60 "About an hour after I drank the sugar . . . I got very sleepy": Annie's blog (Splow27, posted November 17, 2005) accessed November 20, 2005.

62 One Shangri-La dieter wrote, "I would gulp a spoonful . . . gimme more of dat": Annie's blog

(Leftblanc, posted October 14, 2005) accessed November 23, 2005.

63 To learn more about this reaction, I asked Paul Rozin . . . who has studied disgust for more than twenty years: Interview with Paul Rozin, November 7, 2005.

63 "Our subjects have told us . . . are all disgusting," he has written: Paul Rozin, Jonathan Haidt, and Clark R. McCauley, *Disgust: Handbook of Emotions,* 2nd ed. (New York: Guilford, 2000) .

64 An unexpected benefit . . . is that ELOO made their skin feel softer: CalorieLab blog/#comment-690 (Laura, posted November 17, 2005) accessed November 21, 2005.

64 Rozin also pointed out that people are quite poor . . . after repeated exposures: Daniel Kahneman and Jackie S. Snell, "Predicting a Changing Taste: Do People Know What They Will Like?," *Journal of Behavioral Decision Making* 5 (3) (July–September 1992): 187–200.

64 "When I began [drinking olive oil]," she told me, "it was really gross": Conversation with DD, November 2, 2005.

66 Dr. William Jacobs is a professor of psychiatry at the University of Florida's College of Medicine . . . Overeating and Eating Disorders Clinic: Interview with William Jacobs, November 21, 2005.

67 Researchers found that women . . . who drank less than one per month: Mattias B. Schulze et

al., "Sugar-sweetened Beverages, Weight Gain, and Incidence of Type 2 Diabetes in Young and Middle-aged Women," *Journal of the American Medical Association* 292 (2004): 927–34.

67 The nutrition guide . . . has an excellent discussion of their benefits: Walter C. Willett, *Eat, Drink, and Be Healthy* (New York: Simon & Schuster, 2001), 56.

68 A famous clinical trial called the Lyon Diet Heart Study . . . one heart attack: Michel de Lorgeril et al., "Mediterranean Diet, Traditional Risk Factors, and the Rate of Cardiovascular Complications After Myocardial Infarction: Final Report of the Lyon Diet Heart Study," *Circulation* 99 (6) (February 16, 1999): 779–85.

70 One set found that a flavor-calorie association . . . eating the calorie source: Elizabeth D. Capaldi et al., "Conditioned Flavor Preferences Based on Delayed Caloric Consequences," *Journal of Experimental Psychology: Animal Behavior Processes* 13 (2) (April 1987): 150–55.

70 The other set found that a one-hour interval . . . from being learned: Robert A. Boakes and Todd Lubart, "Enhanced Preference for a Flavour Following Reversed Flavour/Glucose Pairing," *Quarterly Journal of Experimental Psychology B: Comparative and Physiological Psychology* 40 (1, Sec. B) (February 1988): 49–62.

71 "I ate *pesto* yesterday": Annie's blog (Masa'il, posted October 3, 2005) accessed November 21, 2005.

72 "Tried this diet for 2 days and I am not as hungry . . . Unbelievable": www.chowhound.com/boards/notfood/messages/64541.html (Adfasf, posted November 16, 2005) accessed November 19, 2005.

72 "This is the first time I have ever left food on a plate": www.freakonomics.com/blog/2005/09/09/freakonomics-in-the-ny-times-the-shangri-la-diet/#comments (Jnyc, posted September 18, 2005) accessed November 19, 2005.

73 "I'm able to feel full after eating about half of what I normally eat": www.freakonomics.com/blog/2005/09/09/freakonomics-in-the-ny-times-the-shangri-la-diet/#comments (Anonymous, posted September 20, 2005) accessed November 21, 2005.

73 "I was a three slices guy; now one slice of pizza is enough": CalorieLab blog/#comment-743 (Leftblanc, posted November 25, 2005) accessed November 25, 2005.

73 "I went to a buffet . . . really bloated afterward," wrote one Shangri-La dieter: Annie's blog (Molly, posted October 1, 2005) accessed November 21, 2005.

73 "I would wake up and crave something to eat . . . through the night, never": E-mail from RJ, November 18, 2005.

73 "I have gotten the best sleep in I can't tell you how long": E-mail from RJ, November 18, 2005.

74 "I would give in and feel bad about myself": Interview with DD, November 8, 2005.

74 "calories of junk—soda, cookies, candy, chips": CalorieLab blog/#comment-743 (Leftblanc, posted November 25, 2005) accessed November 25, 2005.

77 "I still have a lot of mouth-boredom/antsiness": Annie's blog (Masa'il, posted September 30, 2005) accessed November 23, 2005.

77 A few people have reported that the sugar water . . . was ravenously hungry": CalorieLab blog/#comment-688 (Stokely, posted November 16, 2005) accessed November 21, 2005.

Chapter 5. Common Questions

87 Sweetness has the curious feature . . . hungry than when we are not hungry: Elizabeth D. Capaldi, "Conditioned Food Preferences," in Elizabeth D. Capaldi, ed., W*hy We Eat What We Eat: The Psychology of Eating* (Washington, D.C.: American Psychological Association, 1996).

87 I asked Norman Temple, a professor of nutrition at Athabasca University: Interview with Norman Temple on October 26, 2005.

88 In one study . . . eighty times more likely to get diabetes than a person with a BMI of 22 or less: "Type 2 Diabetes and Obesity: A Heavy Burden," a report from *Diabetes UK* (March 2005). At www.diabetes.org.uk/infocentre/reports/obesity _0305.doc accessed November 27, 2005.

88 Another study found that women . . . four times more likely to get diabetes than women with a

BMI of less than 21: Walter C. Willett, *Eat, Drink, and Be Healthy* (New York: Simon & Schuster, 2001), 36.

88 An experiment in Finland . . . reduced their chances of becoming diabetic during the next four years by 60 percent: Jaakko Tuomilehto et al., "Prevention of Type 2 Diabetes Mellitus by Changes in Lifestyle among Subjects with Impaired Glucose Tolerance," *New England Journal of Medicine* 344 (2001): 1343–50.

Interlude. In Shangri-La

90 But here, at Shangri-La, all was in deep calm: James Hilton, *Lost Horizon* (New York: William Morrow, 1933), 142.

90 "Before this, I felt powerless over food": Conversation with DD, November 8, 2005.

90 "It's great to feel like I'm in control of things": Conversation with CM, October 1, 2005.

90 "I never eat the sweets at lunch anymore": Conversation with DD, November 8, 2005.

90 "I just don't have that craving where I'm drawn to the refrigerator": Conversation with CM, November 2, 2005.

91 "[My] weight gain over the years had little to do with being hungry": E-mail from DS, November 14, 2005.

91 "I saw the segment on *GMA* . . . this morning": www.chowhound.com/boards/notfood/messages/64520.html (Laura, posted November 14, 2005) accessed November 19, 2005.

91 "The most enormous difference I can see": E-mail from LJ, August 12, 2005.

91 "I like cookies, and they are available at work": groups.expo.st/art/rec.sport.swimming/5257 (Martin S., posted September 27, 2005) accessed November 16, 2005.

92 "I used to snack all day": Annie's blog (Leftblanc, posted September 30, 2005) accessed November 19, 2005.

92 "My interest in chocolate has dropped dramatically": Conversation with CM, November 2, 2005.

92 "The sugar water seems to be doing away with most of my food cravings": Annie's blog (Zencefil, posted October 16, 2005) accessed November 19, 2005.

92 "Since I have been doing this, my between-meal cravings have all disappeared": Annie's blog (De Benci, posted November 15, 2005) accessed November 19, 2005.

92 "It's just amazing how much my desire to snack has gone down": Conversation with SC, December 15, 2005.

93 "I didn't realize to what extent my nighttime cravings were taking over": Conversation with CW, November 16, 2005.

93 "The best part of it is the snacking is cut out": Conversation with BH, December 6, 2005.

93 "I essentially cut all starches out of my diet permanently": Annie's blog (Molly, posted October 5, 2005) accessed November 19, 2005.

93 "My weakness before the program was junky

carbs": Annie's blog (SFD, posted November 15, 2005) accessed November 19, 2005.

93   "A few weeks ago I would have made a beeline [to the new Starbucks]": Annie's blog (Masa'il, posted September 30, 2005) accessed December 6, 2005.

93   "This Thursday will make 1 full week since I've tried it": www.freakonomics.com/blog/2005/09/09/freakonomics-in-the-ny-times-the-shangri-la-diet/#comments (Anonymous, posted September 20, 2005) accessed November 19, 2005.

94   "I started [six days ago]": www.freakonomics.com/blog/2005/09/09/freakonomics-in-the-ny-times-the-shangri-la-diet/#comments (Jnyc, posted September 18, 2005) accessed November 19, 2005.

94   "I avoid desserts and overeating far more than before the fructose": www.freakonomics.com/blog/2005/09/15/seth-roberts-on-acne-guest-blog-pt-iv/#comments (David Z., posted October 14, 2005) accessed November 19, 2005.

94   "I have used the oil for a week now": CalorieLab blog/#comment-730 (Tina, posted November 22, 2005) accessed November 22, 2005.

94   "Last week a neighbor dropped off a piece of chocolate cake": CalorieLab blog/#comment-743 (Leftblanc, posted November 25, 2005) accessed November 25, 2005.

94   "[Before this diet, I] would sometimes wake up at midnight and eat": Annie's blog (SFC, posted November 15, 2005) accessed November 19, 2005.

95 "I became a night eater": E-mail from RJ, November 18, 2005.

95 "I like to measure time by how long it takes to finish a box of Yodels": Conversation with JC, October 25, 2005.

95 "The diet works, it's easy, I eat whatever I feel like": CalorieLab blog/#comment-737 (Leftblanc, posted November 23, 2005) accessed November 23, 2005.

95 "I do fine during the day—it's in the evening that I have the snacking problem": CalorieLab blog/#comment-704 (Linnie, posted November 19, 2005) accessed November 19, 2005.

95 "No more late-night snacking": Annie's blog (Leftblanc, posted September 30, 2005) accessed December 10, 2005.

95 "The constant thoughts I have about eating have subsided": E-mail from MS, October 27, 2005.

96 "I'm eating to live rather than the other way around": Annie's blog (Molly, posted September 30, 2005) accessed November 22, 2005.

96 "I'm so grateful for not thinking about food all the time": Conversation with DS, November 22, 2005.

96 "I have been able to stop thinking about food": CalorieLab blog/#comment-730 (Tina, posted November 22, 2005) accessed November 22, 2005.

96 "When I do decide to eat, I chose things that are good for me": Annie's blog (Rena, posted December 5, 2005) accessed December 10, 2005.

96 "I am able to make good decisions about how much I need": Annie's blog (Emily, posted December 8, 2005) accessed December 11, 2005.

96 "[Before this diet] I would say I'm not going to eat something sweet": Conversation with DD, November 8, 2005.

97 "I was seeing food as a negative thing because I kept gaining weight": Conversation with CM, October 1, 2005.

97 "When I eat sweets I enjoy it so much more—I savor it": Conversation with DD, October 10, 2005.

Chapter 6. Extra Credit: Six More Ways to Lose Weight

98 "Not sure I look forward to a lifetime of sugar water or oil between meals": Annie's blog (Leftblanc, posted November 23, 2005) accessed November 23, 2005.

99 In *French Women Don't Get Fat:* Mireille Guiliano, *French Women Don't Get Fat* (New York: Knopf, 2004), 5.

99 "French women eat dessert three times a day [at cafés] and they're still thin": Dorie Greenspan, author of *Paris Sweets,* interviewed on *To the Best of Our Knowledge,* February 15, 2004. Available at www.wpr.org/book/030209a.html accessed December 10, 2005.

100 "I think we can say . . . fall outside the Shangri-La Diet": CalorieLab blog/#comment-684 accessed December 10, 2005.

101 *The Flavor Point Diet:* David L. Katz, *The Flavor Point Diet* (New York: Rodale, 2005).

101 "I've been having granola and soy milk for breakfast every day for months . . . Now I'm hungry within a couple of hours": Annie's blog (Jennifer, posted November 20, 2005) accessed November 20, 2005.

102 "The most successful dieters, we've found," wrote Dr. Arthur Agatston in *The South Beach Diet*, . . . a new soup made with every green vegetable he could find": Arthur Agatston, *The South Beach Diet* (New York: Rodale Books, 2003), 43.

102 Yet the husband and wife both drank a lot of Pepsi every day, calling themselves "Pepsiholics": Susan Sheehan, "Ain't No Middle Class," *The New Yorker,* December 11, 1995, 82–92.

103 "I wasn't wanton with my money . . . to splurge on the extra candy bar, the jumbo Coke": Jill Ciment, *Half a Life* (New York: Crown, 1996), 131.

103 When In-N-Out Burger . . . first customer was a college student majoring in health education: Ed Pope, "New Burger in Town," *San Jose Mercury News,* September 7, 1996, 1A.

103 William Jacobs, a professor of psychiatry . . . again, all ditto foods: Interview with William Jacobs, November 21, 2005.

104 Dr. Alan Hirsch, a Chicago neurologist, did a study that suggests this will work: Alan R. Hirsch and Mary Beth Gallant-Shean, "Use of Tastants to Facilitate Weight Loss," paper pre-

sented at the fifty-third annual meeting of the American Society of Bariatric Physicians, 2004.

106 It has an odd name: *food combining.* Typical food combining rules: www.internethealth library.com/DietandLifestyle/Food_combining .htm accessed November 20, 2005.

106 An Italian friend of mine went to a diet expert . . . one type of food per meal: Conversation with AF, November 20, 2005.

107 *New Glucose Revolution:* Jennie Brand-Miller, Thomas M. S. Wolever, Kaye Foster-Powell, and Stephen Colagiuri, *The New Glucose Revolution,* rev. ed. (New York: Marlowe & Company, 2003) .

109 "I just leave off some salt, sweetener or sauce": Annie's blog (Sarah, posted September 30, 2005) accessed November 21, 2005.

110 Timothy Beneke, an Oakland, California, writer, used this idea in a new way: timothybeneke .blogspot.com/2005/09/taste-celibacy.html accessed November 19, 2005.

Interlude. The Blogosphere Tries It

113 After a *Freakonomics* column about the Shangri-La diet appeared: Stephen J. Dubner and Steven D. Levitt, "Does the Truth Lie Within?" *The New York Times Magazine* (September 11, 2005), 20–22. Available at www.sethroberts.net accessed December 16, 2005.

113 "I tried a tablespoon of extra-virgin olive oil yesterday": www.freakonomics.com/blog/2005/ 09/13/seth-roberts-guest-blogger-part-ii (Hal,

posted September 13, 2005) accessed January 4, 2006.

113 "I don't need to lose weight but I must say this sugar water stuff works": www.freakonomics. com/blog/2005/09/13/seth-roberts-guest-blogger-part-ii (Velopismo, posted September 14, 2005) accessed January 4, 2006.

113 "Whoa. Close to zero appetite": www.freakonomics.com/blog/2005/09/13/seth-roberts-guest-blogger-part-ii (Molly, posted September 15, 2005) accessed January 4, 2006.

113 "I've lost 6 lbs. in 5 days, despite eating better than I have in years": www.freakonomics. com/blog/2005/09/18/final-guest-blog-from-seth-roberts (Anonymous, posted September 20, 2005) accessed January 27, 2006.

114 "When I started this, I weighed 226": www.freakonomics.com/blog/2005/09/16/seth-roberts-guest-blogger-finale (Anonymous, posted September 21, 2005) accessed January 27, 2006.

114 "I've lost about 3 pounds in ten days": www.freakonomics.com/blog/2005/09/18/final-guest-blog-from-seth-roberts (Molly, posted September 22, 2005) accessed January 27, 2006.

114 "Your conclusions on fructose sugar are right on the money": www.freakonomics.com/blog/2005/09/15/seth-roberts-on-acne-guest-blogger-part-iv (David Z., posted October 14, 2005) accessed January 4, 2006.

114 "I tried fructose water for 3–4 days and GAINED THREE POUNDS": www.freakonomics.com/blog/

2005/09/18/final-guest-blog-from-seth-roberts (Bonnie, posted September 22, 2005) accessed January 4, 2006.

114 "I've tried the regime for about two weeks now with no results": www.freakonomics.com/blog/2005/09/09/freakonomics-in-the-ny-times-the-shangri-la-diet (Anonymous, posted September 30, 2005) accessed January 27, 2006.

114 "I've been on the diet for three days": www.freakonomics.com/blog/2005/09/14/seth-roberts-guest-blogger-part-iii (Bill Q. posted September 15, 2005) accessed January 4, 2006.

115 De Benci, starting at 185 pounds: Annie's blog (many posts) accessed January 27, 2006. "that I feel I can": posted November 15, 2005.

115 Emily started at 276 pounds: Annie's blog (many posts) accessed January 27, 2006. "It is very interesting": posted November 11, 2005.

115 Julie had little luck: Annie's blog (many posts) accessed January 27, 2006. "I stopped drinking my": posted November 13, 2005.

115 Leftblanc started at 226 pounds: Annie's blog (many posts) accessed January 27, 2006.

116 Masa'il (Hendricks herself): Annie's blog (many posts) accessed January 27, 2006. "definitely irreplaceable so far": posted December 1, 2005.

116 Michelle started at 170 pounds: Annie's blog (many posts) accessed January 27, 2006. "I'm definitely making better choices": posted October 21, 2005.

116 Molly. After two weeks, she wrote: Annie's blog

(many posts) accessed January 27, 2006. "Jeez, this diet makes me": posted October 1, 2005. "So much of what I": posted October 4, 2005. "I lost 12 pounds": posted December 3, 2005. "is a very useful tool": posted December 1, 2005.

117 Sarah's first post said that she had been: Annie's blog (many posts) accessed January 27, 2006. "doing the diet for almost": posted September 29, 2005.

117 SFC started at 184 and over ten weeks steadily lost fifteen pounds: Annie's blog (many posts) accessed January 27, 2006. "This has been nearly effortless": posted November 15, 2005.

118 "Getting the real range of experiences posted": Annie's blog (Masa'il, posted November 20, 2005) accessed January 27, 2006.

118 Robert F. wrote that he had "tried the diet . . . minimal success": Annie's blog (Robert F., posted November 28, 2005) accessed January 27, 2006.

118 Agnostic wrote, "I lost 5 pounds in 3 weeks": Annie's blog (posted December 2, 2005) accessed January 27, 2006.

118 Soon after the *Freakonomics* column, calorielab .com . . . posted a long article about the diet: CalorieLab blog (posted September 21, 2005) accessed January 27, 2006.

119 "I am two weeks into the oil diet": CalorieLab blog/#comment-382 (Paul T., posted September 27, 2005) accessed January 4, 2006.

119 "Separating, through this diet, gimme-energy

hunger": CalorieLab blog/#comment-382 (Paul T., posted October 6, 2005) accessed January 5, 2006.

119 "I am 54, 5´8˝ post-menopausal at 146 lbs.": CalorieLab blog/#comment-263 (Jill, posted September 29, 2005) accessed January 5, 2006.

119 "I have been using the 'Shangri-la' diet now for almost a month: CalorieLab blog/#comment-393 (Alice H., posted October 7, 2005) accessed January 5, 2006.

120 "Have been doing this for 3 weeks": CalorieLab blog/#comment-436 (David Z., posted October 14, 2005) accessed January 5, 2006.

120 "I just have to say it works. I tried it for 2 weeks": CalorieLab blog/#comment-461 (Neema, posted October 18, 2005) accessed January 5, 2006.

120 "I've been following your Shangri La guidelines now for 3 days": CalorieLab blog/#comment-695 (Carmen, posted November 18, 2005) accessed January 5, 2006.

120 "My family doctor recommended that I try this diet": CalorieLab blog/#comment-730 (Tina, posted November 22, 2005) accessed January 5, 2006.

120 "I started this diet on 9/12": CalorieLab blog/#comment-737 (Leftblanc, posted November 23, 2005) accessed January 5, 2006.

121 "Why would I avoid restaurant food?": CalorieLab blog/#comment-743 (Leftblanc, posted November 25, 2005) accessed January 5, 2006.

121 "I can't say enough about the dramatic switch in the way I feel about food": CalorieLab blog/#comment-757 (Stephen M [Ethesis], posted November 28, 2005) accessed January 5, 2006.

122 "I'm a 52-year-old woman, 5 feet tall": CalorieLab blog/#comment-758 (Cheryl, posted November 29, 2005) accessed January 5, 2006.

122 "I have been trying the oil": CalorieLab blog/#comment-1151 (Imtiaz, posted December 23, 2005) accessed January 5, 2006.

Chapter 7. Changing the Rest of the World

123 "I didn't know any English at all . . . for some obscure reason I knew the word *gluttony.*": Khaled Hosseni, talk at George Mason University, Fairfax, Virginia, September 20, 2005 (broadcast on C-Span 2) .

123 "In the year 2001 . . . a woman will have a strong supple and splendid body all her life": Diana Vreeland, www.fashionwindows.com/room__ service/2001/visionaire.asp accessed November 30, 2005.

124 In 1962, a large survey found that 13 percent of Americans were obese: Inas Rashad and Michael Grossman, "The Economics of Obesity," *The Public Interest* 156 (Summer 2004): 104–112.

125 In *Food Fight* . . . television, video games, personal computers, eating away from home, snacking, and "the glorification of overeating":

Kelly D. Brownell and Katherine Battle Horgan, *Food Fight* (New York: McGraw-Hill, 2004), 35–40.

125 Time spent watching TV increased by 45 percent . . . TV watching increased only a little: David M. Cutler, Edward L. Glaeser, and Jesse M. Shapiro, "Why Have Americans Become More Obese?" Working Paper 9446 (Washington, D.C.: National Bureau of Economic Research, 2003). Available at www.nber.org/papers/w9446. This paper also contains measurements of overall activity that contradict the idea that the obesity epidemic was caused by declines in activity.

126 Another reason to doubt . . . low-fat diets produce little weight loss. After a year, most people have lost only a few pounds: Walter C. Willett, "Dietary Fat Plays a Major Role in Obesity: No," *Obesity Reviews* 3 (2002): 59–60.

126 From 1976 to 1996, calorie intake at breakfast, lunch, and dinner increased little, if at all; rather, there was a big increase in snacks: David M. Cutler et al., "Why Have Americans Become More Obese?" See Table 4.

127 "As much as two-thirds of the increase in adult obesity since 1980 . . . fast-food restaurants and full-service restaurants, especially the former," and Figure 7, number of restaurants: Inas Rashad, Michael Grossman, and Shin-Yi Chou, "The Super Size of America: An Economic Estimation of Body Mass Index and Obesity in

Adults," Working Paper 11584 (Washington, D.C.: National Bureau of Economic Research); available at: www.nber.org/papers/w11584. The values for 1962 and 1967 were computed from the U.S. Census of Business assuming that the fraction of food establishments that are restaurants (both sit-down and take-out) was the same in the 1962 and 1967 surveys as in the 1972 survey, which provided a more detailed breakdown.

127 From 1978 to 1996, calories eaten in sit-down restaurants doubled; calories eaten in fast-food restaurants tripled: David M. Cutler et al., "Why Have Americans Become More Obese?" See Table 4.

129 In a 2003 paper . . . (or, to put it another way, a great decrease in food preparation time) from 1978 to 1996: David M. Cutler et al., "Why Have Americans Become More Obese?"

130 Dr. Antonia Demas . . . how schools can persuade students to eat new foods: Interview with Antonia Demas, November 1, 2005.

133 *Totto-Chan:* Tetsuko Kuroyanagi, *Totto-Chan: The Little Girl at the Window,* Dorothy Britton, trans. (Tokyo: Kodansha International, 1982.) "First Prize . . . spinach": page 109. "Get your mothers . . . tastes good": pages 109–110. "He was right": page 110.

135 Cargill, a huge American ingredients company, recently introduced two new sweeteners: Press release, September 12, 2005; available at

www.cargill.com/news/news__releases/050912
__sucromalt.htm accessed November 30, 2005.

Appendix. The Science Behind the Theory Behind the Diet

141 "Am I the only one who thinks this diet might be an enormous hoax . . . perpetrated by the *Freakonomics* guys?": Annie's blog (Jennifer, posted November 18, 2005) accessed December 2, 2005.

141 "I hardly believe it myself": Annie's blog (Leftblanc, posted November 23, 2005) accessed December 2, 2005.

141 "Jaws are dropping around the studio": *Good Morning America* segment, November 14, 2005.

142 Around 1950, a London researcher named G. Kennedy: G. C. Kennedy, "The Hypothalamic Control of Food Intake in Rats," *Proceedings of the Royal Society of London,* Series B, Containing Papers of a Biological Character 137 (889) (November 1950): 535–49.

143 the hormone leptin: Stephen C. Woods, Michael W. Schwartz, Denis G. Baskin, and Randy J. Seeley, "Food intake and the regulation of body weight," *Annual Review of Psychology* 51 (2000): 255–77.

144 "To me this was Newton's apple": Interview with Michel Cabanac, October 28, 2005.

146 To test this prediction, he did an experiment in which subjects lost eight pounds by eating less

of their usual food: M. Cabanac, R. Duclaux, and N. H. Spector, "Sensory Feedback in Regulation of Body Weight: Is There a Ponderostat," *Nature* 229 (5280) (January 8, 1971): 125–27.

146 "This is the first time I have ever left food on a plate at a meal": www.freakonomics.com/blog/2005/09/09/freakonomics-in-the-ny-times-the-shangri-la-diet/#comments (Jnyc, posted September 18, 2005) accessed January 27, 2006.

146 "I'm able to feel full after eating about half of what I normally eat": www.freakonomics.com/blog/2005/09/09/freakonomics-in-the-ny-times-the-shangri-la-diet/#comments (Anonymous, posted September 20, 2005) accessed January 27, 2006.

147 To see if something similar happened with weight . . . "a very flat food," a bland liquid diet: M. Cabanac and E. F. Rabe, "Influence of a Monotonous Food on Body Weight Regulation in Humans," *Physiology & Behavior* 17 (4) (October 1976): 675–78.

148 Around the same time . . . a student in Cabanac's lab named Marc Fantino . . . nutrition without any flavor at all, in other words: Marc Fantino, "Effet de l'alimentation intragastrique au long cours chez l'homme," *Journal de Physiologie* 72 (1976): 86A.

149 Maybe if the food tasted better, they would get fat more quickly, reasoned Sclafani: Interview with Anthony Sclafani, November 11, 2005.

149 This suggested that supermarket food was quite

fattening . . . not just the high-fat foods that made it fattening: Anthony Sclafani and Deleri Springer, "Dietary Obesity in Adult Rats: Similarities to Hypothalamic and Human Obesity Syndromes," *Physiology & Behavior* 17 (1976): 461–71.

150 By accident, he had discovered that rats have a remarkable appetite for a partially digested starch called Polycose: Anthony Sclafani et al., "Sex Differences in Polysaccharide and Sugar Preferences in Rats," *Neuroscience and Biobehavioral Reviews* 11 (2) (Summer 1987): 241–51.

150 Sclafani and a colleague set up an apparatus . . . directly into a rat's stomach whenever it drank: Anthony Sclafani and Jeffrey W. Nissenbaum, "Robust Conditioned Flavor Preference Produced by Intragastric Starch Infusions in Rats," *American Journal of Physiology— Regulatory, and Integrative Comparative Physiology*, 24 (1998): R672–R675.

151 In the following years, Sclafani and his colleagues did hundreds of experiments about flavor-calorie learning: Anthony Sclafani, "How Food Preferences Are Learned: Laboratory Animal Models," *Proceedings of the Nutrition Society* 54 (1995): 419–27.

152 He did so much great work . . . about whether sugar causes obesity: Interview with Israel Ramirez, October 27, 2005.

152 "It is widely believed," the paper began, "that

consumption of sucrose may predispose human beings to obesity": Israel Ramirez, "When Does Sucrose Increase Appetite and Adiposity?" *Appetite* 9 (1987): 1–19.

153 The right amount of water could *double* the weight gain: Israel Ramirez, "Diet Texture, Moisture and Starch Type in Dietary Obesity," *Physiology & Behavior* 41 (1987): 149–54.

154 Maybe the saccharin would make the food taste better so the animals would eat more of it: Israel Ramirez, "Stimulation of Energy Intake and Growth by Saccharin in Rats," *Journal of Nutrition* 120 (1990): 123–33. "First evidence": page 132.

INDEX